SOUL'S HARBOR

True Adventures of *Medic-13*

Based on actual events

NICHOLAS BLACK
with
IAN FEDEROV

Author's note: The stories described in this work are based on actual events. The names of individuals, locations, and various details have been changed to protect their anonymity.

* The opinions and techniques in this book are those of the authors. Any medical procedure or treatment mentioned may not be current. One should always adhere to the most current AHA ACLS (*Advanced Cardiac Life Support*) and ATLS (*Advanced Trauma Life Support*) techniques.

www.NicholasBlackBooks.com

www.SoulsHarborProject.com

Copyright information:

Library of Congress Catalog Number:

ISBN 10: 0-981-94940-6

ISBN 13: 978-0-981-94940-6

Printed in the United States of America

Three Spears Publishing.

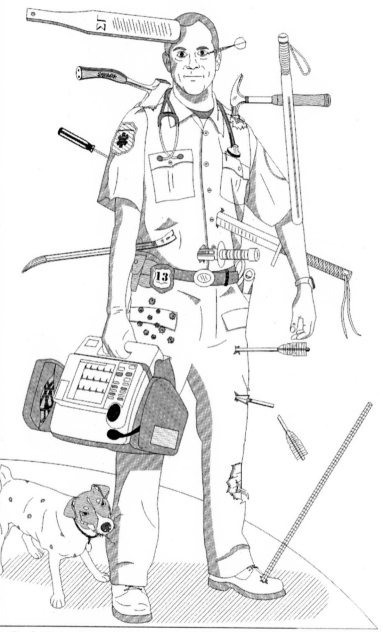

"Medic-13" © Ian Federov 2008

Contents

For Leslie

OTHER BOOKS BY NICHOLAS BLACK:

FICTION
PURG
BURNING HEAVEN

SEE JACK DIE.
SEE JACK HUNT.

SODOMY CAT
THREE WISE MEN
CONTRACT KILLER (WITH JIMMY DASAINT)

NON-FICTION
THE LAST AMERICAN MERCENARY
WALKING GHOST

Soul's

HARBOR

True Adventures of *Medic-13*

FOREWORD

My friend, Nicholas, asked me to tell him, at length, about my old job. It's my fault. I began most of our conversations with, *"When I was a medic..."* Even though I've spent many years trying to forget these ghosts, I'm still walking around with them in my head.

"People need to know this stuff," he said to me. So, I figured, this is my chance to get 'em out in the open. To release them once and for all. Clean out my closet. That was until I recalled the delivery of that baby. That one I'm gonna keep.

A wise man once told me that if I found a job that I wouldn't mind doing for free then that is the career I should pursue. Well, who wouldn't want to race around to rescue folks in need, meet and work with intelligent people, and never get bored? There are a number of reasons to work in EMS (Emergency Medical Services). I figured those were mine. Simple enough.

I began my seven year career in EMS by taking a college course which I thought would be an easy 6 credits. It wasn't long before I knew it was my calling in life. I continued on to the paramedic program. I also attended firefighter school. You can never have enough education in the area of life saving. I gave it all I had and I got much in return.

Some good and some bad.

This work is highlights of my career for the intent of telling a story. Many EMS professionals may find some similarities to there own experiences. I do not claim a dominance in my tales to others or boast. God knows we hear enough of that. I just want to entertain and give an account. Perhaps make you smile. There's an old Russian proverb that goes something like, *'People like us don't have friends, not like us'*. So, people who don't work around this environment have a hard time understanding what happens at a scene. And they have an even more difficult time understanding what we go through before and after the call.

People should know EMS is not always full of hero stuff. It is all too often we run head long into this way of life with benevolence and spunk. Then when we least expect it we become flotsam of a society that is out of control. Chewed up and spit out. We can no longer return to what the multitude deems normal. Not after years of greedy hospitals, miserable paychecks, long hours of over-time, and patients who don't want our help.

And yet, when the call comes, we shrug and head to the ambulance.

If you're working in EMS pat yourselves on the back and remember to take care of yourself. Better yet, pat your partner on the back. They probably need it more after putting up with you.

—Ian Federov

Prologue

A few years ago . . .
Springfield

Imagine falling off of a roof and landing on a barbed fence post, right through your thigh. Picture sliding your left hand across a table saw, leaving your fingers on the 2x4 as your brain tries to make sense of it. Ponder tripping backwards and cracking your head on the corner of the swimming pool as you slide into the water unconscious.

Try and imagine that feeling when your windshield is exploding in slow-motion, shards of glass racing toward your face as your body is jerked around like a rag doll, pieces of metal and plastic twisting around you. Imagine that being my life.

We get called to the scene of a *'man down!'*

That's all they say.

That's all we know.

Could be a million different things that brought this man down. You can't rule anything out in this business because the most improbable, unlikely of scenarios is usually what we get stuck with.

In her typical, static-laden voice, the dispatcher tells us to head to Trinity First Baptist. So we're thinking, *church people*. And for the most part, church employees are relatively grounded, respectable types. These are the kind of people you can count on. These are the folks that barter with St. Peter to get us past the Pearly Gates, so they're usually trustworthy.

So whenever they say someone is *down*, it's got to be seriously.

The dispatch was explicit when she explained that the callers were *"excited"*. And if you think about it, there's a million horrible things that could happen at a church. Think of all the hard, pointy phallic, guilt-ridden edges that somebody might stumble upon. And get past the physical dangers, and consider all the emotional and psychological baggage that church goers tote around on a daily basis. The kind of people that go to church, need to be at church. They need saving.

In my mind I'm picturing divorced guys toting shotguns, angry teens carrying knives, sharpened crucifixes in the hands of jealous lovers, the out-lash of a demonic possession . . . who knows?

As we pull up to the medium-sized, white-painted wood church I realize something isn't right. The whole scene is an instant contradiction. The Christians who ran up to us as we stepped out of the ambulance were frantic and worried, hands and eyes darting around like they'd seen Satan naked in the shower or something equally disturbing. They're all going nuts.

The firemen and other safety workers, on the other hand, were smiling, almost on the verge of tears as they held back their laughter. I see hands over faces.

Shoulders bouncing up and down. People literally biting down on their bottom lips so they don't collapse into laughter.

"You've got to help him!" a young woman wearing a blue sweater nearly screamed. I could see sheer panic in her eyes.

"He's not talking right!" a young man said, his round glasses fighting to stay in place, what with his nervously sweating face. He could be on soap operas, this guy.

" . . . I don't even think he's breathing. He's got to be *dead*, by now!" another woman said through her fingers.

"Hurry up!"

We go around the side of the church, stepping across the carefully manicured lawn and we see the fire Captain. He's knelt over the patient. We approach quickly and he turns to address us. And he utters just two words,

"Billy . . . Angel."

As our shoulders and heads collectively sag, he apologizes to us for not warning dispatch sooner. I hear my partners whispering the kind of profanity that should guarantee them a hot seat in hell. And I'm just kicking the grass at my feet.

Feeling betrayed, we all drop our gear, shoulders sloughing, sighing frustratedly. Because, really, we all know we just got duped. Don—my boss, otherwise known as *Medic-23*—turns to go and speak with the Christians. He rolls his eyes to me as he heads toward the group who are still pretty much *shitting-in-their-pants* anxious.

Picture a guy with loose-cropped red hair, a thick red mustache, and a squinting look on his face as if he was always staring past the sun at something. He had a bit of a stomach on him, but he wasn't obese to the point where he'd get his own reality show.

Why *Medic-23* got this task is that he's the most calm, unexcitable person on the face of the earth. He routinely arrives at horrible scenes of violence and unspeakable carnage only to nod slowly to himself.

One time, when a guy's head was on the hood of his car, several feet from his body, *Medic-23* looked at us, shrugged, and said, "Shooooo." That's it. Nothing more. Not an "Oh my God!", or a "Holy shit!". No, just a *shoooo*. It didn't even warrant an exclamation mark it was so subtle.

Most people, including me when I first came to work with him, attributed his calm under pressure for a lack of adrenalin in his body. We figure he just ran out years ago. I mean, how many grotesque scenes can your mind wrap itself around before they all seem trivial and tame? You get desensitized in this business. And he's been working as a paramedic for over 30 years, so he's seen it all . . . twice.

But the reality is, he keeps his composure under the most awful of circumstances due to his mental problems. He's got wires crossed in that big head of his. Somewhere in the grey matter there are dendrites and axons and neurons that are fizzled and broken. So, in situations like this, he's the guy who usually goes and talks to frantic, screaming church people.

What that means is that I'm the guy who gets to work on Billy Angel. I sigh, shake my head a few times, and kneel down. I'm looking at the curiously clean *Branson, Missouri* t-shirt, a pair of dirty jeans, an overcoat that is so soiled and disgusting that it might be a dumpster liner, and what look like a pair of cotton gloves with the fingers cut out.

He's got the classic bum look, with the signature bum scent—a mixture of cigarettes, piss, hamburgers, feces, and spoiled milk. And now that I consider it, most bums have the spoiled milk smell, above all others, that instantly identifies them. And I've never even seen a bum drinking milk, but that's neither here nor there.

His skin is leathery and looks like it's been stained with *Thompson's* all-weather sealant. The capillaries in his face are all busted, especially around his nose. It's like some wrinkled road map. On his wrists are a variety of brightly colored plastic medical bracelets from the many hospitals he's been a recent guest at.

And he'd either been drinking *Listerine*, or his own piss. Or maybe he'd been drinking his own piss from a *Listerine* bottle . . . it's hard to nail down exactly which.

Oh, yeah, and he's absolutely fine.

One fireman in the background says, "Hey, didn't we send him to Fayetteville?"

And now is the point where I need to make a small admission. We had been getting so many calls for Billy Angel in the past couple of years—an average of twice a day or more—that we all engaged in a rather petty conspiracy. All the police, paramedics, firefighters, and various other safety services pitched-in to buy him a bus ticket to Fayetteville.

Somebody thought that maybe he had family there. *Maybe.*

So we scooped him up, delivered him to the bus station, made sure he got on the bus, and wiped our hands clean of the biggest system abuser in Springfield. We thought that our troubles were finally behind us, safely tucked away behind state lines. We all figured that the quagmire that is Billy Angel was now somebody else's problem.

But no. Here he was, staring up at me with his vacant blue eyes. You could see the yellow of jaundice in the whites of his eyes due to his failing liver. This, unfortunately, is also rather characteristic of bums.

At first glance you can't help but feel sorry for the guy. You almost want to pick the guy up and hug him. Tell him things are going to be alright. That there's help. But all that fades quickly.

"Hey there, Billy," I said. "It's been a while, huh?"

His face gets wrinkled and mean, "You, you think you're better than me? I didn't call you. I went to college . . . you piece of shit! Fuck you."

My hands that could be hugging him, they could just as easily be punching the cheap vodka out of his face.

"Okay, Billy, nice to see you, again, too," I say. I've seen him a hundred times in the last year, and he still doesn't recognize me.

"Why can't you just leave me alone? You people are always messing with me." Then his eyes seem to fidget a bit, " . . . hey, uh, you got a cigarette?"

The police department actually ran his prints after he got caught stealing liquor from a drive-through liquor store. It turns out that he did in fact go to college. He used to be an agent with the Drug Enforcement Agency. Word is, he got busted in some bribery scandal while he was working undercover on a drug-trafficking case. Once word hit, his wife and family left. He became an alcoholic, and it was all downhill from there.

"Are you hurt anywhere, Billy?" I asked, glancing over the myriad wounds on his body, trying to identify the new from the old.

"I didn't even call you," he says, glancing at the church dumpster that he occasionally calls his bed. "Dickhead," he murmurs.

Strange thing about Billy is, he's just intelligent enough to *really* piss you off. Like he's got a gift for it. He kind of knows what people are thinking, just by reading them at a glance. Remnants of his old life as a DEA agent, maybe.

I ask him, "Do you want to go to the hospital?" I'm not so much feeling bad for that guy as I am following protocol. I have to ask that question, by law.

"Hell no, I don't want to go to the hospital. I'm fine. Fuck you, you fucking asshole!"

I laugh to myself. You can't let him get to you. Or at least, you can't let him *know* he's getting to you.

He's like a shark in the water, if he smells so much as a drop of emotional blood, he'll attack.

"Well," I reply, "then you need to sign this refusal so that the cops can take you to jail."

His eyes grow wider by a factor of three as he clutches for his chest, "I . . . can't . . . breathe!" Like I said, the guy knows how to use the system.

I nod, "Okay, Billy. I'll be taking you to Medical Control today, unless you have another preference?"

He's just doing the grabbing at his imaginary chest pain thing, now. Really selling it. And while he's nodding at me, everyone else is rolling their eyes, looking up at the sky.

In the ambulance, on the way to the hospital, I notice the multi-colored bracelets again. "Billy," I ask carefully, "what were you at the hospital for?"

This is important so that we don't accidentally treat him with any kind of emergency medicines that might decide to have a sparring match in his blood stream with hospital meds.

He pulls out this folded piece of white paper, handing it slowly to me. It was on official *Fayetteville Fire Department* letterhead. And beneath the official address and bold print, there were big, angry, handwritten letters. No signature to be found.

And it said,

Screw you guys!   Keep your trash in Springfield.

That letter went straight to our station's bulletin board for all to enjoy. The bad nickel that is Billy Angel had returned to haunt us.

Looking at the eerily clean *Branson* t-shirt, my mind was doing all sorts of back flips trying to put it together. I asked him what had happened.

He half-burped, then swallowed something that must have been awful, answering, " . . . oh, uh, when I got to Fayetteville the fire department put me on a bus to Branson, where my girlfriend lives." And then he smiled, licking the underside of his lips in a gesture that still gives me shivers to this day.

She must be *special*, I said under my breath.

"Huh?"

"Then what, Billy?"

He stares off somewhere near the ceiling of the ambulance, "My girlfriend and I had an argument, so I caught a ride back to Fayetteville."

" . . . and then?"

"Oh, uh, the fire department people put me on another bus back to Springfield." Then he laughs at me, turning his nose up, "They were *professionals* . . . unlike you dicks!"

"Shut-up, Billy," I said. "Just . . . just pretend you have chest pains until I get rid of you."

Then I get on the radio, "**Medical Control, this is Metro-Three, we're inbound to your facility with,**" and I swallow, " . . . **William Angel.**"

And there's this awkward pause before I hear a reply. And, following this audible groan, I hear, "**Copy that Metro-Three, we'll have his room ready.**"

When I look back at my career, and the perverse things I experienced, his name invariably pops-up over and over. He's got so many ridiculous stories that surround him that it's hard to determine what I can tell you, and what I need to try and forget.

Like the Tramp Camp riots.

Or the night he got raped.

The day he got blown-up.

All of it is pure gold. The kind of stuff no writer could ever imagine actually happening. But this is the kind of thing we deal with on a day to day basis. It's not the only thing, it's just one of the more animated parts.

When cars flip over, or industrial machinery explodes, or a hungry tiger escapes the zoo, or some clown with *daddy* issues pulls out a shotgun full of hatred, I might be the guy they call.

Hi, I'm Medic-13, and I'll be your savior this evening.

1

ORIENTATION

March 16, 1993
Thursday, 7:30 am . . .

Welcome to Springfield, population 200+ thousand.

Springfield city is located in southwestern Missouri, near the James River, at the northern edge of the Ozark Highlands. It sits just north of the Table Rock Lake area. It was settled in 1829, but its growth and development were rather slow unitl the period of heavy westward migration, when pioneers were attracted to its convenient location near several major land routes.

During the American Civil War, the city was besieged and held by Confederate forces for a few months after the Battle of Wilson's Creek (August 10th, 1861; fought 11 miles to the south). They were eventually expelled by Federal troops in February of 1862.

The legendary "Wild Bill" Hickok lived in Springfield and scouted for the Federal Army. He was acquitted there of the murder of Dave Tutt.

A rival community, North Springfield developed as a result of an extension to the Atlantic and Pacific

Railroad in 1870, but in 1887 both Springfields merged.

To give you an idea of the kind of people you are dealing with on a daily basis, keep in mind that their economic mainstays are dairying, aluminum boat and barrel manufacturing, and various other agricultural ventures.

This city is, and I hate to admit this having dated many women from here, a redneck town if there ever was one. I won't go so far as to call it *White Trash USA*, but I sure hear the phrase being thrown around when the town is mentioned . . . even by some of its less than sociable citizens.

It's in the numbers. When more than 50 percent of your workforce is employed by fast food restaurant chains, you might have a problem. This is an entire society raised on partially-hydrogenated vegetable oils and artery-clogging trans fats. They're happily obese, and anyone that tells them any different must be stupid.

However, for all the bad dieting, risky mating practices, and suspect behavior, you also have a rare strain of kindness in these small-town folk. They care about each other intimately in a way that people from a bigger city can't relate to.

Where I grew up, in south Chicago, people would step over a dead body to grab the newspaper. Nobody cares about you except your mother. And dad would tell you that after he belted you. Once, when I was younger, a guy was threatening to jump off a building near our house. Traffic was jammed in every direction, pissing off all kinds of people.

And the first words of advice to this suicidal man came from the mouth of a dark-skinned taxi driver who yelled, "Jump you fuckin' fairy! Ain't you got the balls?"

Springfield was different. People looked at each other. They cared what was going on in their community. If a road had potholes in it, there were meetings and arguments and bake sales. When a girl got pregnant, everyone knew about it as fast as a whisper can spread. People went to church, as a social event. Kids went to the same schools that their parents attended. There was a connection with each other that they all shared.

Despite their decidedly hillbilly underpinnings, they were decent people, with strong religious morals and ties. They have a host of educational institutions —*Evangel College* (1955), *Central Bible College* (1922), *Baptist Bible College.* We've even got the *International Headquarters of the Assemblies of God Church* here. So, we're neck deep in the lord almighty.

And for me, this was all an incredible culture shock.

I did my EMT training at a nice community college. It looked like an easy class that I could take to steal some credits. Six months, that's it. I mean, how difficult could it be to get cats out of trees, and rescue grandmothers who'd fallen down flights of rickety old stairs?

The next course I took was the EMT-Paramedic (Emergency Medical Technician-Paramedic). That course was over a year long. And much more difficult than I had expected. The way they explained it was, anything you can do in the first few minutes in an Emergency Room, you'll be able to do after completing the EMT-P. And they're not kidding. I saw things, touched things, and learned things that I had no idea were a part of emergency medicine.

So here I am, fresh out of school, bright-eyed and hungry for action. I put in applications all over the place, and land a job in downtown Springfield. Maybe it wasn't my first choice. Or my second, third, or fourth. But it was somewhere in my list.

My first day on the job I show up at a place that is supposed to be the headquarters of *Metro Emergency Medical Service* (Metro-EMS). But the place I was looking at, through the windshield of my old Ford Ranger, didn't look anything like what I imagined Metro-EMS Headquarters to be. This place was like a big red house with three huge garage doors on the side.

I drive around the block several times, checking my directions over and over until I see a large slope-side ambulance race by. I follow it back to this unlikely building where I park and head toward the front door.

As I entered, a rather frumpy, uptight group of women eyed me suspiciously, waiting for me to speak. Right about the time I was going to introduce myself, one of the women pushed her coke-bottle glasses up her huge nose, saying, "You Stubbs? The new guy Stubbs?"

"Yes, ma'am. I'm Daniel Stubbs," I said. "I'm supposed to meet Rick Parker for my—"

"That's a strange name," one of the other women said, turning her chair toward me, "Stubbs. What kind of name is that, anyway?"

"I'm Irish."

"Stubbs doesn't sound Irish," the woman with the bionic glasses adds.

A younger woman, maybe in her early twenties, she folds her arms across her chest, "Irish names are like *O'Reardon* or *O'Malley*. But I don't know about Stubbs. That doesn't seem Irish."

And as both my family name and my ancestry are getting picked apart by women that wear skirts and blouses the colors of old Chevys, a short, chubby little man walks in the other side of the room. He looks up at me and his face seems to slacken. I'm not sure if he's happy to see me, or frustrated that I actually made it.

"You're Stubbs, right?"

"Yes, sir."

One of the women says, "He claims to be Irish, but we're not so sure."

This chubby guy was very spirited and energetic. More than I'd expect for an obese man. He almost vibrated he was so excited. "Daniel," he said, looking down at a clipboard in front of him. He glanced up, " . . . so?"

So . . . what?

"So, are you Irish, or aren't you?"

I laughed, "Uh, yes. I'm most certainly Irish."

Ricky looked over at the women who didn't look convinced. Even the younger woman—who as I study her closer is quite attractive in an accountant-secretary kind of way—isn't sold on my Irish blood.

"Are any of you ladies Irish?" Rick says as he waves me to him.

As I'm walking between rolling chairs and small desks the women are shrugging, no.

"Well, then," Rick says with grin, "since none of us are Irish, how the hell would we know one way or the other?" And then he looks at me, nods a couple of times, "Daniel Stubbs, welcome to Metro EMS. Never mind these women up front, here. They still think we faked the moon landings."

And as they begin to voice their protests he walks me into the Day room—where people watch television, play video games, or gawk at pornography. Then he led me through the kitchen—refrigerator, table, microwave. As he gave me some of the basics we passed the sleeping quarters—consisting of six small bedrooms, one for each medic on duty.

We passed by a supply room that had the drug box and all of the medical supplies. This place, so far, had a rather worn-out, almost tired look to it. But it was also comfortable. Something between a house and an office.

And it was quiet.

I don't know what I had expected. This place reminds me of a fire station. And I guess that's a pretty fair analogy considering that we're both—paramedics and firemen—meeting up at most of the same locations. All of our pagers go off at the same time.

Rick, as he's leading me around, pointing things out here and there, I'm picking up on something anxious and almost neurotic about him. He speaks very fast, with almost a used-car salesman's cadence and tone. I could imagine him pitching financing rates and haggling over percentage points at any moment. But that fast-talking way was just how he communicated. He would be good at reading that legal information at the end of car commercials.

He takes me by a large room which he refers to as the Training Room. That's where we would have all of our continuing education courses, First-Responder classes, staff meetings, CPR courses, and other procedural meetings that would come up from time to time. It was full of chairs and tables and presentation equipment.

There were mannequins and training aids, and a curious black muck near the upper edges of the walls. He sees me eyeing the walls near the ceiling and assures me that it isn't poisonous mold. In fact, he told me that twice, which left me a little less comfortable.

Then we made our way into the garage area. When you first walk into the garage area you are in the wash bay, where the ambulances—referred to as 'units'—drive through and hose out all of the blood and guts from the previous call.

As I'm looking around I notice a fidgety looking man approaching me. Rick says, "Wonderful," then turns to me, "this is going to be your partner, Tim Wheeler."

I take a good look at Tim. He's fat. He's got a bad rug on his head. And he's got dodgy eyes that look to have seen something the rest of us keep missing. As he approaches, Rick whispers through clenched teeth, "He's a Vietnam Vet." And the way he says it, it's more of a warning than a salute.

When he makes his way around the bay to us, we shake hands. The best way I can describe it would be shaking hands with a dead octopus. Imagine slimy tentacles for fingers. A cold, almost fishy texture to his palm. Kind of listless and creepy. I can already see myself not wanting to be left alone in a small room with this guy.

"I'm Tim Wheeler," he says, his eyes glancing around behind us.

"Daniel Stubbs."

"Stubbs?" he says. "What is that, Polish?"

Rick laughs, walking me to a small group of para-medics that are fiddling with a clock radio. I meet a bunch of guys and the mood is really informal because it's a private company.

Rick then hands me off to Tim, who takes me around to the units that are parked and ready to go. It's explained to me that I'll be in the back of the unit, in the jump-seat, as a 3rd rider while I'm training. That's my on-the-job training position. While I ride and assist on the calls I'll be introduced to various hos-pital employees (ER nurses and Doctors), nursing home administrators and nurses, firefighters, and police officers.

They're introducing me to the fraternity of para medicine. As far as patient care, everything that I learned in college takes precedence. I have all the tools to save lives, but I don't know anything about actually doing it in the field.

When we got back from the unit they hand me a Medical Protocols and Procedures book. The thing is about 3 inches thick, and Tim tells me to read-up because I will be tested first thing in the morning.

They hand me a pager and a radio and we made our way into the day room where we sat down and started watching cartoons. The whole time I'm waiting for the 'training' to begin. But, as I soon learned, you get your training during the calls.

"What do we do now?" I asked Tim.

He was chewing on his thumbnail with a kind of psychotic zeal that made me wonder how he's not in a mental institution. "We'll go and check the unit in a minute, *Beavis and Butthead* is almost over."

For real?

2
SUICIDE SOLUTION

Headquarters
Metro-EMS garage

After *Beavis* finished trying to light his farts on fire with a lighter, we made our way back out to the garage, and to the ambulance that we would be driving. We don't have an assigned vehicle since they are constantly in and out of the shop for repairs.

We head to the second of three large bays where a large white slope-side Ford Econoline, Powerstroke diesel-turbo is waiting. The words *METRO-EMS* are painted in bold black on the sides, on the front doors, and on the bumper as well.

"Got to familiarize yourself with the unit," Tim said, opening the back doors.

Part of that familiarization involves checking the O^2 source, the outside lights, the diesel fuel levels, making sure all of the sirens are operational—typically 5 out of 10 aren't functional.

We then check the side doors for the various equipment: the Thumper (to manage chest compressions) and the oxygen tanks that power it, the Jaws of

Life (a hydrolic-powered pry), the C-collars and towel rolls, the scoop stretcher, and the KED (Kendrickson Extrication Device)—a half spineboard used for securing patients.

Then we do an inspection of all the packs: the Oxygen pack, the Pediatric pack, the Obstetrics pack, the Burn kit, the Trauma pack, the Cardiac monitor pack, the Narcotics box (for which the crew chief has a key), and the splints.

All of this stuff is inside each and every unit, just waiting to be used. And all of it must be inspected every single time you go out on a call. Once that's done, and any items are replaced or replenished, we take out all of the dirty linen and medical waste that has not been disposed of from the last call. In some cases, the last call could have been hours or even a day ago, so you might have quite a robust mess on your hands.

Etiquette would say to clean your unit after use, but this is often overlooked or neglected after particularly difficult calls.

Anyway, after all of this has been done, and you're checked-in, you take the unit around the wash bay for a nice cleaning. You give it the full rub down: all surfaces, windows, and even the wheels and tires get a shine. Then it's time to sit on your ass and watch more cartoons, or play *Nintendo*. You might, at a bigger station, go and run errands—collecting backboards and other miscellaneous equipment that stayed with the patients you delivered to the different hospitals.

But not us, and not right now. No, we're just watching a mouse take aim at a cat with a shotgun. For the next few hours I'm thinking, this is the greatest job, ever. And that's when we hear the call coming over all of our radios . . .

12:44 pm . . .

"Springfield Dispatch to Metro-EMS . . . we have an attempted suicide, gun involved, police are en route."

All of the sudden we spring out of our chairs, sprinting for the unit. The crew chief—a young, quite attractive, 22-year-old girl named Samantha—was already starting the engine. Tim raced off, and by the time I got there, they're already rolling. I had to pull some *James Bond* maneuvering just to jump inside before she left me!

"Nice of you to join us, Rookie," Samantha said as I clawed my way to the jump-seat.

My old, fat, burn-out, Vietnam Vet partner, Tim is giggling like a chubby little pig. When I was in the day room, one of the other paramedics, a guy named Henry, told me that Tim wears the hair piece to cover a napalm burn that left horrible scaring on his head. The government actually gives the guy a yearly stipend to purchase new wigs. Thing is, though, he's so cheap that he keeps the cash and uses the same wig. It makes him smell like *Lysol* disinfectant. It's more than spooky.

We settled ourselves in the unit, and as I got to talking to my partners I realized that they were as different as two humans could possibly be. Samantha was graceful, calm, and a consumate professional. Tim was slow, clumsy, and easily flustered and excited.

She responded, "Metro-EMS to Springfield Dispatch . . . Metro-five en route, ETA three minutes. Request status of police on scene."

"Whenever you hear a gun is involved," she said while driving and handling the radio, "you ask for cops."

After what seemed like a long, bumpy ride, we arrive at the scene. There are several police cars and a firetruck parked with their lights flashing. My heart is really pounding!

Suddenly, we hear the dispatcher break the silence, *"Springfield Dispatch to Metro-five . . . police and fire on scene, weapon is secure. Caller is in contact with police. They're waiting for you inside."*

We jump out of the unit with Samantha ordering me to pay attention and listen to what she says. "Don't think," she tells me, "just do."

We're at a large, rather intimidating apartment complex that looks to be something between section-8 housing and the doorway to hell. We enter a dark, dank, seedy, wet, and downright disgusting cave of a place that seems as if it is composed of manure and rotting stucco. There are bits of metal here and there, and I feel like I need a tetanus shot already.

We're going to the second floor. Three groaning steps up, and I want to spray-paint *my* brains all over the wall. This is no way to live. We made our way up, escorted by a fireman who seems hellbent on leaving us behind. Like he's got somewhere else to be.

After a silent, dimly-lit hallway that is devoid of color we are welcomed into an explosion of sound and excitement. People are running in every direction like those bouncing rubber balls that you get in gumball machines.

The room we enter is full of smoke. And not the pleasant scented candle kind. No, this was the blue, lung boiling smoke with the *Marlboro Man's* signature on it.

Police are trying to secure the family, who are puffing on their cigarettes, quietly dividing up their share of the estate. They look as interested as a bunch of janitors at a high school football game.

Samantha grabs all the relevant information from the police and firefighters.

How long has he been down?

Who started CPR?

She then grabs her radio and calls for a second ambulance.

The patient is laying on a bare matress that is on the floor. No sheets, no pillows, just pools of sticky blood next to the aged yellow piss stains. And a firefighter is performing CPR, but with no effect because the matress is cushioning the body so that the compressions are useless. The guy's body is just bouncing up and down.

"Move the patient to the floor, please. You're not getting chest compressions on that surface," she says forcefully, but calm.

She drops her airway pack and kneels down at the head of the patient. She's checking for the three most important things:

Airway.

Check.

Breathing.

Check.

Circulation.

Check.

And as she's checking him, she commands Tim to set-up an IV, and crack the seal on the Drug box. She finds no pulse, to go along with the bullet hole in his head.

Tim seemed lost and confused. And it was that point that I had to step-in. I think Tim was stuck back in Da Nang, taking artillery fire or something. He was completely out of his tits.

Samantha intubated the patient—lowering a scope into his throat and inserting a tube down his throat. Then they hook up a BVM (Bag Valve Mask). She's so quick and practiced that the tube goes right in, and she makes it look easy.

Anyway, I straddled the patient and began to handle the chest compressions. Tim, at this point, can only be trusted to operate the BVM, which consists of little more than squeezing a plastic bag. He's trying to keep in sync with me doing the compressions, but it's nearly impossible. I compress, he squeezes, and we're each doing our own thing.

A fireman then pulls out the *Lifepack-10* (Cardiac monitor, Defibrillator/ Pacemaker) with the big defibrillator pads. One goes on the lower left side of his chest, the other goes on the upper right, just below his shoulder. They call them *fast patches*, and once they're on you can see basic heart activity. He has a rhythm of some sort, then she's shocking him.

His pulse is still not there. So we keep working on him.

Samantha then went to task setting-up an IV on the patient's right arm. Next thing, we're pushing fluids and drugs in to him so fast that I don't know what's happening.

During all of this madness, a fireman is still trying, in vain, to plug the quarter-sized entry hole, searching frantically for the exit wound.

We get the patient secured onto a backboard— *packaged-up*—and the six or seven of us around the backboard lift him. We race him out of the apartment, across the dark hallway, and down the rickety, unsteady stairs. We're in such a hurry, in such a confined dark space, that one of the firemen gets his whole pinky finger pinched off along the way. But we didn't find this out until much later because there was so much chaos that he didn't even notice until we were loading the patient into the unit.

There's no way to explain the kind of lunacy and madness that are sewn into every minute spent during a call. I couldn't tell you how much time went by until I looked at when the call was received and when we left. Time doesn't work in a linear fashion when there are so many people doing so much to keep a person alive.

Minutes and hours and seconds get all garbled and confused.

Moments later we are slamming the doors of the unit shut, Samantha beside me while we continue CPR. The second ambulance finally arrives as we are pulling out of the parking lot. They'll have the job of cleaning up the scene and recovering all of our leftover medical gear and equipment.

Now we're en route to the hospital.

One of the firemen is driving while Samantha communicates with the hospital, administering medication, reassessing the patient. I'm still just handling the chest compressions.

Tim is maintaining the BVM, squeezing occasionally, and oxygenating the body. He's also making sure that the endotracheal tube is still in place.

And he is *technically* performing his job requirements, but he's also in the throws of a major freakout! I think *Victor Charlie* is taking pot shots at him right now, as he winces sporadically to unseen things.

And that's when the patient's stomach contents suddenly come up, spraying all over Tim. Luckily, Samantha's tube keeps the patient from aspirating spoiled milk and *Mad Dog 20/20*—the kinds of cocktails that poor suicidal bastards drink before they pull the trigger.

I'll be honest, I'm not sure what's more kind, saving him, or letting him die. To wake-up back to the world he lived in, I'm not sure that isn't cruel and inhumane.

Something seems to confuse Samantha while she's on the radio, "Metro-five to St. John . . . "

"St. John . . . go ahead Metro-five."

"Metro-five to St. John, we're currently inbound to your facility with a Priority-one trauma code. Twenty-two year old, male patient with a self-inflicted gunshot wound to the head . . . " then she looks at the patient, squinting at something, " . . . thirty-eight caliber."

The fireman who's driving, he says, "Hey, lady, it's the other way around. He was thirty-eight, and the gun was a twenty-two caliber pistol."

Samantha shook her head, toggling her radio, " . . . gunshot wound to the head, we're sure of that! Excessive bleeding." She then informs the hospital that all ACLS (Advanced Cardiac Life Support) protocols are being followed. That's important so that they know we did everything by the book.

"Our ETA is one minute!"

Thing is, we all know that the reality is that this patient, our Priority-1, he's a corpse, now. But once we start CPR, they're alive. Nobody dies in an ambulance. Ambulances are for the living.

Hearses are for the dead.

So, we can't call death until the patient gets to the hospital, no matter how dead they really are. Doctors *pronounce* death, we announce it These are the legalities of death.

And this . . . this is my first day.

3
SLAUGHTERHOUSE RULES

January 6th
Thursday, 11:52 am . . .

"Springfield Dispatch to Metro-EMS . . . we have a medical emergency at the Pennington Slaughter House. Caller says 'broken leg' and the man is conscious."

I've got half of my first bite of a delicious chicken sandwich in my mouth as my supervisor's familiar scratchy voice graces the airwaves saying, *"Metro-EMS to Springfield Dispatch . . . Metro-three is en route."*

And now I'm spitting out my delicious, fresh chicken sandwich with lettuce and tomatoes and just the right amount of mayo. I'm doing this because Don has volunteered my unit's services. See, Don knows where I like to eat lunch. He knows how fast I drive, and even the kind of music I enjoy listening to.

He knows everything.

As it turns out these days, I'm Metro-3. So this is our call. And it really sucks because I've been to the last three calls this morning, but my unit happens to be accidentally closer than anyone else's, so I win the ambulance lottery. Or lose; it kind of depends on your perspective.

Sitting across the formica-covered table from me is Tim, eyeing his sandwich like it's a cleverly disguised explosive device. It's been over a year since I started working with Tim, and he's still messed-up. Vietnam seems to be very much a part of his waking moments, haunting his days as well as his nights. I guess he eats to compensate. Well, he compensates a lot, because he's fatter than ever. I feel like I'm gaining weight just being near the guy. His shadow weighs more than me.

"Tim!" I say as I stand, "that's not the enemy."

He looks up at me, then uses his knife to tap on the top of his sandwich bun a few times. Oddly, no ticking noises can be heard.

"We've got a call, Pennington Slaughter House," I remind him.

"Shit," he says as he scoots out of the booth, "that can't be nice." And as he removes himself from the friction between the plastic booth and the table top, I realize that our days as partners are growing short. It can't last. He's such a nervous, worthless piece of trash. He's completely unreliable. He is *not* the guy you want jabbing a large-bore needle in your arm and administering drugs into your bloodstream.

We head out to the unit and I get in behind the wheel. I'm a crew chief these days. Turns out I'm pretty good at this type of work. I'm not as calm and collected as Medic-23. But I don't crap in my pants and freak-out like Tim, either. I'm just the right mixture of neurotic and desensitized to be a good paramedic. Stuff still bothers me like the next guy, but I wait until the shift is over to consider it.

I legislate times for empathy and emotional catharsis. But that time is not during working hours.

We take off, and less than eight minutes later we are pulling up in front of the Pennington Slaughter House. This place smells like death from about two miles away. As we pull into the parking lot there is a large group of dirty old men wearing knee-high boots, cover-alls, plaid shirts, and those mostly plastic-billed caps with farm equipment company logos—you know, the basic redneck ensemble. And right now, they're all waving their arms as if we might miss the place without their help.

"Shit," Tim says under his breath.

Yup.

Tim and I park and get out of the unit, following these men back to where they corral the cattle. It's this dark, caged pit. And I don't know how the whole system works, but I have this feeling that this area is the last place that animals enter *alive*. Off to the side, a young man is laying on his back in a mixture of straw and dirt and liquid cow manure. This is the most horribly dirty and disgusting place you can ever imagine being. To work in such a place . . . forget about it.

The guy on his back is moaning, his right leg bent 90 degrees the wrong way—kind of off to the side of his leg, against the proper motion of the knee joint. I kneel down, looking at what seems to be several large stomp marks. They're all over his chest and body. So, in addition to the completely fractured lower head of the right femur, he has probably got other broken bones from where the cows did the Riverdance on him.

Behind me, this skinny guy with a few extra chromosomes says, "We tried to straighten it for ya', but we ain't no doctors. Besides, Billy wouldn't let us touch it!"

Tim circles around the patient in order to hold in-line stabilization of the head, but on his way around he takes a bad step and rolls through the manure, sliding and crashing to a stop at the feet of some perplexed workers. And they must see people fall in this place all the time because they don't even laugh.

I sigh, shaking my head as I look down at the man, "Billy, we're here to help you out, okay? When my friend picks himself up he's going to hold your head while I ask you a few questions. We have to make sure they didn't hurt your neck."

Billy looks to be in his early twenties, still young and without the signature wrinkled leathery face of a life spent working in a place like this. He looks scared and I'm trying to calm him down so that he doesn't panic. I'm not worried about shock because that's pretty much a phantom.

Let me explain. Shock is a failure of the circulatory system to supply sufficient blood to peripheral tissues to meet basic metabolic requirements for oxygen and nutrients, and the incomplete removal of metabolic wastes from the affected tissues.

Shock is usually caused by a hemorrhage or overwhelming infection and is characterized in most cases by a weak, rapid pulse; low blood pressure; and cold, sweaty skin. Depending on the cause, however, some or all of these symptoms may be missing in individual cases.

There are several varieties of shock: Physiological shock (from cardiovascular disease), Bacteremic shock (caused by various bacterium: *Escherichia Coli, Proteus, Pseudomonas,* or *Klebsiella organisms*), Anaphalyctic shock (allergic reaction as the result of foreign material into the bloodstream), Cardiogenic shock (progressive decline after acute and severe cardiac damage), Neurogenic shock (autonomic nervous system shock cause by interruption of blood volume or nerve severance in lower body), Insulin shock (diabetics), etc.

And then there is Psychogenic shock. This is the kind that you see somebody crying "come back, come back!" in Hollywood movies. You know, the man is down, slowly dying in the final scene, and the attractive girl is kneeling beside him, screaming for him to keep his eyes open. This type of shock is the fainting kind.

We also refer to it as *pussing out!*

In a nutshell, blood pressure falls, the skin gets cold and sweaty, and the pulse rate increases. A decrease in the amount of blood flowing to the brain leads to light-headedness and loss of consciousness. But that doesn't mean the person has been lost to some magical barrier from which death takes its final hold.

So, as a paramedic, I'm not worried about a guy fainting. I'm worried about the underlying cause. And in Billy's case, he's relatively aware. His pulse is strong. That makes it easier for me to ask him the kinds of questions that need asking in a situation like this.

What I am most concerned about is Hemorrhagic shock. See, if Billy has a severed femoral artery as a result of his fracture, then he could easily bleed internally. And quite quickly. Arteries are under serious pressure so they will forcefully squirt blood. Venous injuries are less serious because at that point the blood is coming back to the heart, and has much less pressure.

My first move, after Tim has gotten in-line stabilization, is to straighten the leg using a traction splint. I basically position it as straight as I can, getting Billy as comfortable as possible under the circumstances. Then what we do is called "packaging" the patient.

This involves putting him on a backboard. The first concern is the neck, which we stabilize with a C-collar. Then we place towel rolls on the sides of his head so that we can tape his forehead and the C-collar to the backboard itself.

The final touch is to secure the chest, the hips, and the legs of the patient with straps that look a lot like seatbelts by the way they clip and fasten on the sides.

While all of this is going on, I'm getting the explanation of what actually happened by a group of guys whose average IQ is probably in the lower to mid '60s.

Apparently, Billy was in the caged area, trying to help along the traffic flow of the steers. He was urging them to a choke point where they line up single file to bid farewell to the land of the living, ending up on a burger plate at some point. As he was pushing one of the steers he got kicked in the nuts.

As you can imagine, a hoof from a steer will put any man down on the ground. Billy hit the floor only to be stomped repeatedly, and nearly trampled as the steers went wild.

A guy at the top of the shoot, who goes by the name Flea, saw Billy fall down. He yelled immediately for the others to move in and clear out all the steers. At some point, after the animals were gone, they realized that they couldn't 'pop' Billy's leg back into place, and somebody with a 3rd grade education called 911.

We lifted Billy carefully and placed him on a gurney, headed for the parking lot. As we rolled out to the unit, several men were walking with us, assuring Billy that everything was going to be alright.

"Don't worry, Billy, we killed that steer that done this to you!"

"He's dead, Billy," another man assured him. "That some-bitch is dead!"

And I thought that was a curious way to emotionally comfort their fallen comrade, since all of those animals were just minutes away from being slaughtered anyway. I guess that's society's need for revenge or something. I'm no shrink, though.

As we loaded Billy up in to the unit, I decided to let Tim stay in the back with the patient. They both smelled like all flavors of crap, and I was on the verge of gagging.

"Metro-three to Springfield Dispatch . . . Metro-three transporting one," I said, trying to only breathe through my mouth. That's the key. Don't use your nose. Because if you do, it's like you're eating whatever you smell.

I immediately rolled down all the windows, put the unit into drive, and we left the Pennington Slaughter House without lights or sirens—*non-emergency*—on our way to the hospital.

And I know, beyond any doubt, that I'm not going to get to eat lunch today. If by some chance I do, it certainly won't be a burger.

4
CONCRETE PROOF

May 1st
Sunday, 5:26 pm . . .

"Springfield Dispatch to Metro-EMS . . . injury accident. Twenty-ninth and Range Line."

Tim and I just finished a non-emergency transfer. I grab the radio, "Medic-thirteen to Medic-twenty-three . . . we're available at St. John's."

"Copy that."

Don answers quickly, *"Metro-EMS to Springfield Dispatch . . . Metro-three and Metro-five are en route."*

The reason he's sending out two units is because 29th and Range Line is a high traffic area, and we imagine it's going to be dangerous. It's just on the other side of a railroad bridge and people have a tendency to come off of the bridge hauling major ass!

Tim is with me, bitching about not getting his promotion to crew chief. His hair piece looks more artificial than ever, like a house cat stapled to his head, and he smells like disinfectant, again. It's like some kind of cruel joke.

"Tim," I say, "you failed your medic exam four times." The guy's not even fit to apply *Band-aids*. Some kid watching *ER* could be a better service to the wounded than him.

"Well . . ."

"Well, nothing!" I bark as I switch on the lights and sirens. "You shouldn't even *be* a medic. Maybe this line of work isn't for you. Maybe you should just do the dump-truck thing full-time."

He doesn't answer, but I can see he's plenty angry. He's fuming under his skin, his teeth clenched tight, his jaw muscles shifting from tensed to *really* tensed. I expect to see smoke come out of his ear canals any second.

He has a part-time job driving a dump-truck. I've been pressuring him to take it up as a permanent career so that he doesn't risk so many lives. He's just a terrible medic, and a liability. To add insult to injury, he's still resentful that I promoted past him for crew chief, a position for which he thought *he* deserved.

Turns out you have to be more than a warm body to promote. You actually have to be a capable paramedic, not just show up for work on time.

Let me tell you something else about my shell-shocked partner: He hates it when I drive. He is scared of speed. Absolutely, out-of-his-tits, scared shitless. And I drive like a bat out of hell each and every time he's riding with me. I floor it every chance I get, and in my peripheral vision I can see him stabbing his foot into the floor, trying to hit some imaginary brake pedal, while his hands claw deeper and deeper into the seat cushions.

Every time I see him shiver or squirm as a result of my driving habits, I have this overwhelming urge to laugh maniacally, but I don't succumb to it. I don't want him to know it's all by design. I'm basically trying to scare him into quitting.

This is an indirect form of playing *Chicken*.

So, right now, we're at speeds that rival Mach 2, on our way to the accident scene.

As we arrive on the scene we see several police cars spread out, keeping the through traffic under control. There are also two firetrucks—a pumper and a rescue truck. The rescue truck has a fascinating bit of history attached to it. Ironically, it used to be a beer truck. The fire department purchased it, refurbished it to get rid of the beer smell, and voila.

The police have shut down two lanes of the four lane highway. And one of the officers waves me off to the side. I notice our other unit—Metro-5—arriving from the other direction at almost the exact same time.

Once on a scene I have to gather information as quickly as possible. I have to determine who I need to help first. The more serious the injury, the more in need of assistance they are.

And the story I get is this: A white Toyota pick-up came speeding over the bridge, toward a *Southerland's*— home furnishings, lumber, etc.—at which the driver and passenger were employed. The problem came when the entrance they intended to use was occupied by a large cement truck. The Toyota was going *Dukes of Hazzard* fast, and it met the cement truck at the rear quarter. You know, where all the cement is?

Toyota vs. *Cement truck.*

Winner: Cement truck.

Well, the guy in the cement truck barely even felt the accident. But the occupants of the Toyota were messed-up something serious. As I walked up to the passenger side an unconscious man was being extricated by firemen. He had on a C-collar, and he was big.

In the bed of the truck was the driver. He was so big he must have bounced forward and then rebounded backwards, exploding through the rear glass. His body somehow ended up in the bed of the pick-up. There were firemen holding in-line stabilization, waiting for us to get here.

A quick note on in-line stabilization. When you're doing it, the act of carefully straightening the neck and head is accompanied by your inspection of Airway. And that's the A of the ABCs (Airway, Breathing, Circulation.)

The fireman holding the passenger suddenly yells, "The passenger is coding! The passenger is coding!"

There was blood everywhere. Both of this guy's legs are broken and twisted so much they looked like *Jello.* Like bags of chunky red sauce. His face was lunch meat. Blood everywhere. Bits of bone and plastic and vinyl and glass and hair all mixed into a kind of accident soup.

No signs of life.

I know, for certain, that the passenger was not just *coding!* He was dead.

Dead dead.

In my assessment, the passenger is a goner. The guy in the bed might have a chance, so that's who we need to focus our efforts on. It sounds cruel and heartless, but it's the reality of the situation.

So Tim, in his brilliance, starts CPR on the passenger as I got to the driver. The driver was the only viable patient. That's the sad truth.

But here's the problem with what Tim has just done. Once you start CPR, you can't stop until they get to the hospital and a doctor calls time-of-death. So what he has inadvertently done is commit us to the DRT (Dead Right There). And that means we've lost valuable time and resources that need to be dedicated to the only viable patient—the driver.

For reasons beyond my comprehension, the other ambulance crew took to helping Tim with the dead passenger. They might as well have been practicing on a mannequin. Maybe he called them over, or . . . I don't know. But I'm working like crazy to keep the driver alive.

My patient was unconscious, with broken legs, a host of severe head injuries, not to mention all the stuff I can't see beneath the blood. And there is blood all over the place. We have to package him up as quick as possible, getting him out of the truck.

We get him quickly onto a backboard and lower him to the rolling cart. Within seconds we are racing him toward the unit where we can actually work on him. It's just a fireman and I, both of us trying to do the same thing—keep this guy alive.

Once we get to the unit I get the patient intubated, hand off the BVM to the firefighter to continue breathing. I slap on two fast-patches and get the monitor up and running. He's got a Sinus Tachycardia—that's a really fast heartbeat. I start an IV and then glance around for my idiot partner, Tim.

"Goddammit, where's Tim?" I gripe.

The fireman, who's ready to drive me to the hospital, says, "He's workin' on the other patient. The DRT."

We can't wait. I glance up, "St. John's . . . let's go!"

I slammed the back doors shut and we're out of there. As we start rolling we hear the radio, "*Medic-thirteen . . . you're partner is running behind your ambulance.*"

I grab my radio, keying-up, "You can keep him!"

Then, addressing dispatch, I say, "Metro-three to Springfield Dispatch . . . transporting one to St. John's. We'll be running hot!"

"*Metro-three to St. John's . . . five thirty-six.*"

The fireman turns his head slightly in my direction, letting his foot off the gas, "What about your partner?"

"Who?" I reply as I study the monitor.

"You don't want to pick him up?"

I point my thumb back through the small window in the back of the ambulance where my partner's wobbly figure is shrinking and disappearing. As he's running, the wind is picking up the front of his toupee, and he's starting to wobble unsteadily.

Next thing I know he takes a tumble, rolling ass over elbows down to the pavement. What a retard. As far as I was concerned, he was dangerous. This guy routinely sticks endotracheal tubes down people's esophagi. He inappropriately touches female patients when he's alone with them in the back of the unit. He makes wrong drug calculations.

He's useless.

The guy killed people, in my opinion. He is a sorry piece of garbage. Human trash. That's the *best* thing I can say about him.

"That guy?" I say. "I don't even know that guy. I don't even know where he got the uniform."

And with that the fireman laughs, guns the throttle, and we head to the hospital. Later, after it was all said and done, I heard that the passenger was in fact *dead* dead, on the scene. My patient, the driver, he eventually made a full recovery.

The city even put up a stoplight at the accident scene, just before that bridge. In this town, somebody has to die horribly before a stoplight gets put up. That's Springfield's version of evolution, I guess.

5
HEAD-ON

May 13th
Friday night . . .

"Springfield Dispatch to Metro-EMS . . . we have a two-vehicle injury accident on Highway forty-four. Rural-fire is already en route."

Medic-23, our supervisor, answers, *"Metro-EMS to Springfield Dispatch . . . Metro-three is en route."*

And this is the part where I sit up groggily, blinking several times to get the sleep out of my eyes. Metro-three, that's us. I get up quickly, putting on my boots and jacket as I race out to the day room where I know my new partner, Ernie, will be.

Sure enough, he's sitting at a table, completely prepared, finishing off his fifth bag of *Peanut M&Ms*. Ernie is big. He stands six-foot-three, weighing in at over 350 pounds. He's got those big porky-pig cheeks, with thick round glasses and a mustache. He has a host of health problems because he is so big.

He's the kind of guy that I figure we'll have to eventually answer a call for. Ernie is always a breath away from a massive heart attack. Once he gets going, wheezing and puffing, you just know his days are numbered.

But then that's just the physical side of Ernie. The thing about him is, he's always ready for a call. He lives for it. He always has all of his gear prepared. He's the most enthusiastic paramedic I've ever met. He wants to answer every single call that comes over the radio. And it's tiring working with a partner like that because it means that *we* have to answer every call. Boring or not, he wants it. Morning, noon, or midnight, he's game.

Most people say, "Ernie, he might be big, but he's got more heart than any other paramedic alive."

And no matter how close you are to the unit, once a call comes in, he's there, raring to go. If he's driving, the unit is always started and idling. If he's the passenger, he'll have his clipboard out, writing things down.

So we head out, flip on the lights and siren, scream through the town at breakneck speeds until we're out of the city limits. The whole time that we're driving, we're hearing all sorts of radio traffic. It's all just blackness and wig-wags—the side-to-side strobing effect of the lights dancing off of pavement and trees.

I get on the radio, "Metro-three en route . . . please put LifeFlight on standby."

An excited guy comes over the radio, "*We have a ten-fifty, J-four!*" Which translates to a motor vehicle accident, *with* fatalities.

I'm handling radio traffic as Ernie drives. I get a full description of the accident—numbers of patients and types of injuries sustained—and then I call for a back-up unit to respond, and I also make sure that LifeFlight is in the air.

See, any accident that involves a fatality instantly raises the threat level because anyone involved could be on the doorsteps of death themselves. They may look and seem okay, but since they were right next to a dead person, there is a very real chance they sustained similar physical damage.

About 10 minutes later we see a Christmas Tree—the assortment of different emergency lights and sirens of all colors—up ahead like a brilliant beacon in the otherwise pitch blackness of the night. All traffic is stopped and the area is aglow with flares and emergency vehicles and bright strobe lights.

Off to the right there are guys out in the field, setting up an LZ (Landing Zone) for the LifeFlight medical transport helicopter.

And then we see the collision. It looks like two dark piles of twisted metal and broken glass. It's difficult to imagine that it ever used to be two different vehicles. The moment I see this, my brain trying to make sense of it, my heart just sinks. I know, for sure, that there have to be dead people.

Lots of them.

Ernie and I jog over to the firemen who are trying desperately to extricate the patients. One man had self-extricated—ejected during the crash—and was laying nearly 50 feet away from the accident.

And this was the story: A vehicle with five passengers crossed the path of a vehicle with two passengers, coming in the opposite direction. A head-on collision ensued. There were beer cans in what was left of both vehicles, right along side the dead bodies.

In the car that had carried the five passengers, three of them were dead. All we could see was a bloody mangled arm, long black hair, and some fleshy bits—all of it encased in bent metal. This person, that we were looking at bits and pieces of, they were already dead, so there was no reason to worry about extricating them at this point.

Both vehicles were pouring out radiator fluid and oil from beneath, and the interiors were filled with blood. With the lights from all the vehicles, it might as well be daytime. There is too much detail. This is the wrong way to see death.

This is like looking at high-definition, technicolor carnage. This madness represents a weird moment in time that doesn't conform to the path these people were supposed to follow.

It's one bad instant.

Less than a second from laughter to the abyss.

As the first medics on the scene, we take over scene management from the fire department who had created a makeshift triage center. The triage—a French word meaning 'to sort'—is basically an area used to assess the different priority levels. These are: Priority-1 (immediate life threats), Priority-2 (potential/possible life threats, to be monitored closely), Priority-3 (walking wounded, can wait for medical treatment), and Priority-4 (dead, mass-casualty, imminent death, not to be treated).

One fireman was taking care of the man who had ejected from the vehicle.

Right now, everything is happening at the same time. We are making order out of chaos so that we can save *somebody*.

Of the three surviving patients, two were Priority-2s and one was a Priority-1. We immediately sent the Priority-1 to the LifeFlight that had landed within two minutes of our arrival on the scene.

We packaged the Priority-2s and loaded them into the unit. And let me describe the environment; there are people everywhere. There are tons of volunteers helping us move the patients to the unit. Both volunteer and full-time firefighters jogging back and forth.

Wreckage and smoke and lights and noise . . . and blood.

As we headed out, the volunteers stayed behind with the bodies—referred to as DRTs—until the coroner arrives. Their injuries were "incompatible with life". These people weren't *almost* dead or *maybe* dead. No, they were *dead* dead. Mutilated beyond any question or doubt. The only way to ask them questions now was to use a *Ouija* board.

One of the firemen was driving the unit while Ernie and I were in the back with the patients. We're looking down at two teenage girls with their whole life ahead of them . . . maybe. Hopefully. Now they're fighting for their futures while my partner and I follow our ATLS (Advanced Trauma Life Support) protocols.

They get the works: Large-bore IVs, EKG, high-flow Oxygen, and a full body assessment. We're seeing them as machines that have to be repaired. Not as humans. Not as delicate young kids who were having a fun night out. There isn't enough time to consider that this young woman in front of you is dying.

You have to go!

Fix the machine.

Fix the leak.

There are no mistakes in an ambulance. There can't be. Even in this confined space, big Ernie is a professional. There are no *missed IVs*, or *ooops*, or *I can't find a vein*. What's taking over now is training and experience and adrenaline, and they're all working together to make you more efficient. You don't have to be God; you have to be better.

Airway.

Breathing.

Circulation.

Then check it all again.

Because if we screw up, these kids are *dead* dead! And like I said, ambulances are for the living.

That kind of power and influence over the course of a human life is something that can attract you to this field, or destroy you. The emotional baggage and psychological pondering that usually follows, it's saved for later. When the adrenaline is exhausted and the call is over, that's when you're left with your thoughts.

These girls, they'll become human when we're cleaning the clotted blood out of the back of the unit while the Rolling Stones are playing lazily in the background of the garage.

That's when you reflect on the frailty of life and the ease at which death finds us. Luck and fate and all of that. Catharsis is the aftermath.

We got them to the hospital, dropped them off to the emergency room staff, and waited. Those three surviving kids . . . they lived. And I'd rather remind myself of that, than of the four kids that didn't pull through.

My mind only has enough room for so many ghosts. And at some point you just have to start forgetting them. Old phantoms replaced by the younger, newer, more visceral images.

6
TRAMP CAMP RIOT

October 24th
Monday, 3:26 pm . . .

"Springfield Dispatch to Metro-EMS . . . we have a medical emergency. There's been a stabbing under the Seventh Street Bridge, industrial area. Officers are on the scene."

Oh-no! I'm thinking as I grab my radio. Seventh Street Bridge can mean only one thing . . . the Tramp Camp!

I head to the closed bathroom door where Ernie is backing one out. He got a hold of some bad burritos earlier, and he's been making us pay for it ever since. I hammer my fist against the door, "Pinch it off, Ernie. We've got a call to the Tramp Camp!"

I then lifted my radio and answered the call, "Metro-EMS to Springfield Dispatch . . . Metro-three is en route."

I can hear him shuffling around, probably not making any attempt to wipe. His own radio keying-up as he struggles to pull his pants on. Everyone in the city can now hear Ernie pulling his pants up. I so hope he doesn't comment on the damage his burritos have caused while he's broadcasting live across the city frequency.

This kind of thing actually happens more than you'd think. People, especially heftier people, will accidentally toggle their city-wide frequency without knowing it. And, of course, they start talking about things that they shouldn't be.

Subjects like: who's going to get fired, who's sleeping with who, what doctors are sleeping with what nurses, how attractive that last overdose patient looked with her shirt off. You know, the kinds of discussions that are supposed to remain between partners. Last year a guy learned that his wife was cheating on him with another paramedic under similar circumstances. Anyway, no good can come of it.

Right now, Ernie is broadcasting the final throws of a turd to the entire city.

I have learned from experience to back away from the bathroom door when he's in there because at any moment the 350-pound freight train is going to bust through there and haul ass to the unit. And trust me, you *have* to get out of his way when he's coming through!

Nothing comes between Ernie and his ambulance.

Sure enough, he explodes through the door. As I run behind him I yell, "You've got an open mic, Ernie! All of Springfield just heard you take a dump."

"Dang-it!" he barks as he makes his way to the driver's side of the unit. Six seconds later the engine is purring as I pull myself up into the seat.

We *light'em up*—initiating all the bright spinning lights—and hit the sirens, and off we go!

The Tramp Camp is right around the corner, no more than four city blocks from our station, so we're there almost instantly.

Long ago there were two large shipping and receiving warehouses with a large space between them through which railroad tracks ran. In this in-between area the trains used to be unloaded and loaded. It's covered with a thin metal roof that extends between both buildings, probably 30 or 40 feet high. The companies have long since departed, the tracks no longer exist. When industry moved out, the bums moved in. But this creates what is affectionately known as the Tramp Camp.

Under the cover of the old metal roof, 25 or 30 homeless people have created a makeshift home. This was an open-air house, but it was a place where they could survive the elements.

In the center of this open space was a trash can fireplace for cooking, hand warming, and whatever else it is they do to stave off hypothermia on a routine basis. It can get incredibly cold down here. The wind blows by with that howling chafe that makes you shiver just hearing it.

Surrounding the fireplace are decrepit old couches and end tables that seem to have been dragged out of a dumpster. They form a loose circle. This is the *living room*.

Beyond the living room were matresses and more trashcan fireplaces. They really could use some drapes to brighten up the place. Oh, and everything is a shade of earthy brown. The color of things masked with soil and decay.

As we arrive on the scene, there are at least five police cars, one firetruck, and a bunch of scattered vagrants that looked plenty pissed that we were in their business. Ernie and I jump out right after the police assure us that the scene is secure. They lead us to the stab victim. Ernie pulls off to check out the other homeless guys, setting up a Tramp Camp triage.

The patient was laying on one of the garbage couches with his hands over his stomach. And almost instantly Billy Angel appears, letting everyone know that *he* understands how to handle the scene. He tells us not to worry, that he's checked out the injury and that the guy only has a scratch.

"I'll take care of it," Billy Angel informs the rest of the bums.

We brushed off Billy and assessed the status of the victim. Looking at the guy we could tell he's been beat on repeatedly. His ears and cheeks and eyes were all swollen and scratched. He looked like somebody had opened up a 12-pack of *whoop-ass* on him.

I look at this ball of clothes and bruises, and I ask him, "Sir, can you tell me where you're hurt?"

All gruff and angry, he replies, "Can't you see . . . it's right here." And then he removes his hands.

"Did you get stabbed, sir?" I ask, trying to figure out if this is the right guy. I notice, under the camouflage of a battered face, that this is Robert Salter. He's not as infamous as Billy Angel, but he's well known none the less.

He looks at me with this incredulous glare, "Are you stupid? Can't you see the knife? It's still in there."

And sure enough, as his hands move and his body shifts a bit, I see the steak knife buried deep into his abdomen. The first and main concern in a stabbing of this nature is whether a hollow or solid organ has been punctured.

Since everything about the guy smelled like blood, feces, and ammonia (from old urine), I was worried that a solid organ such as the liver or spleen might be punctured. People that get drunk for a living have abnormally large livers. Thus, they become bigger targets for stolen steak knives.

Livers are extremely vascular, and blood loss due to a laceration is my main concern. We have to secure the knife in the abdomen for the hospital Emergency Department staff to remove at a later point. We do not remove the knife! Never pull out the implement that is stabbed into you! The knife or arrow or piece of glass or shard of metal might be the only thing preventing uncontrolled internal bleeding; or do more internal damage by cutting and lacerating on its way out. Leave it in place.

As we begin to use trauma dressings to secure the knife in place, the guy starts to crash. He stops talking to us, becomes rather incoherent, as his skin turns flush and clammy.

I yell to Ernie, "This one is a *load-and-go!*"

He can barely hear me because the bums are getting louder and more agitated, starting to scream at each other. This place is a homeless powder keg. Some old toothless hag is actually punching Ernie in the back, but he can't even feel it through his rolls of fat.

Cops are running around doing nervous crowd control as things continue to escalate. The shouting gets louder and the bums seem to be turning violent. It's time for us to get out of here.

We package him up as quickly as possible. C-collar, towel rolls, backboard in place, we hurry him to the safety offered by the back of the unit. Behind us the fighting has officially begun. It looks like a scene out of *Gladiator*, only with frantic police and withered old bums throwing the punches and kicks.

At any moment we should be able to taste the sting of mace in the air.

We have a fireman driving for us as I start to intubate. Ernie quickly starts the IVs—one in each arm due to the rapid loss of fluid. See, another thing about alcoholics is that they imbibe so much alcohol that their blood is thin and anemic—their blood doesn't clot well, if at all.

So once they start bleeding, they just keep on leaking until they're bleeding out Ringer's Lactate (balanced salt solution, for fluid resuscitation). Ringer's is a little better than normal saline; well, until you see it pouring out of your patient.

When they're bleeding pink, you know you've given them enough.

I've got the defibrillator pads on Robert's chest, watching the monitor closely. It looks like he's got an SVT (Super-ventricular Tachycardia), which is an abnormally fast heart rate. Pretty much, the heart is getting ready to leap on out of his chest.

SVT usually precedes V-tach (Ventricular Tachycardia) and V-fib (Ventricular Fibrillation) which usually equals death. In V-tach the heart is just a quivering mess, not pumping any blood.

We're tumbling down the road, bouncing all over the place. Firemen, as gifted as they are, aren't the best of drivers. Luckily, the ceiling is padded because we're hitting it repetitively with our heads and shoulders.

Ernie gets on the radio to the hospital while I manage the BVM squirting 100% oxygen into Robert's lungs.

"Metro-three to Medical Control . . . we're inbound to your facility with a Priority-one trauma. Fifty-six year old, male trauma patient. Stab wound in the upper left abdominal quadrant. Vitals are: thready, pulse over two-hundred, blood pressure sixty by palpation, respiration's assisted at eighteen-to-twenty a minute. The monitor shows SVT, rate of two-forty . . . "

Ernie pauses for a half-second to catch his breath, swallowing, "We've stabilized the bleeding. Patient is intubated, breathing with BVM at one-hundred percent O-two. Patient is fully immobilized. We have large-bore IVs, bilateral A.C.'s running at a KVO rate. We have an ETA of five minutes. Do you have any questions or orders?"

"Negative, Metro-three . . . maintain ATLS protocols, we'll see you in five."

After everything is said and done in the emergency room, old Robert Salter pulls through. Ernie and I are right outside the emergency room, at the ambulance entrance, cleaning out the clotted blood and bio-hazard medical waste. You don't rush this part of the job.

We're carefully pulling all the *sharps* (needles) out of the seat cushions where we stick them in the heat of a call. That's better than dropping them to the floor to get stepped-on. There's no telling what kind of horrible disease and rot is under the vinyl skin of these cushions.

When we finish cleaning the unit, we sit back and have a quiet cigarette. Right now, we're just riding down the adrenaline rush. We're listening and laughing to the radio traffic concerning what would later come to be known as the Tramp Camp Riots.

I turn to Ernie, "Did you know that old Robert in there is a retired firefighter?"

"Really?"

"Yeah," I say, "from California."

Ernie takes a long pull from his cigarette, the smoke drifting slowly out of his nose and mouth as he says, "You know, Danny, you and I . . . we're just one or two paychecks away from being *him*." He nods to nobody in particular, studying the blue smoke for sagely answers.

" . . . just a paycheck away."

Later on we learned that the Tramp Camp Riots started when our man Robert insulted the integrity of one of the local ladies—indistinguishable from the local men. That led to shouting, pushing, punching, probably a fair amount of spitting and slobbering, and eventually stabbing.

As things happen, a day later a dead body turned up. This lead to the city fencing off the entire area and making it off-limits to everyone. That left the bum community with only two choices: drink somewhere else, or stay sober and go to Soul's Harbor.

7
WATER HAZARD

Emergency Medical Services Appreciation Dinner
Saturday evening . . .

Throughout the year we have different dinners, ceremonies, and get-togethers for the Emergency Medical field. The big one, however, is at the end of *EMS Appreciation Week*. There's a large semi-formal dinner that brings us all together, usually sponsored by a local hospital. The hospitals throw these little shindigs to win favor among the EMS workers.

The theory behind this is that we have a *choice* of which hospital we'll be bringing our broken patients to when we're racing around trying to keep them alive. As if, with one hand on a gaping wound, and one fumbling for an IV we're trying to figure out which hospital threw the better party, and therefor should get our patient.

Which is *complete* nonsense, because you don't have time for all that. But as long as they keep an open bar, we'll keep showing up to these events.

By semi-formal I mean that most of us dress quite appropriately in nice clothes. Key speakers might wear fancy suits. Rednecks would be wearing jeans and boots, with ridiculously large belt buckles, even though we all know they've never competed in a rodeo.

The audience consists of firemen, police officers, paramedics, doctors, and nurses . . . especially nurses. The dinners are usually a quiet evening in a large banquet hall with people receiving awards and commendations as we all picked apart whatever the overpriced meal was.

The spirits flowed quite freely, and you can imagine things deteriorating into a kind of controlled chaos. For the most part, though, people were on their best behavior. You see, you don't want to make a scene at an event like this because anyone in the room might be your next chief, or supervisor, or rescuer.

The people in this room, if I ever keel over and have a heart attack, one of them is going to be getting the call. Another of them is going to arrive and secure the scene. Somebody else that might be sitting three seats away is going to be the girl that intubates me, putting a tube down my throat so that I can get oxygen.

So all of us are linked to each other, whether we realize it or not. Right now I'm sitting at a large round table with about 10 or 12 other people. Some guy named Art is at the podium right now giving a mind-numbing speech about a helicopter that crashed on the highway, or a car that crashed into a helicopter on the highway, or a highway built on top of a car that looks like a helicopter. Truth of it is, I can't pay much attention. Art, he has a kind of monotone speaking voice, and I think I'm being lulled into a coma the more I listen.

Most of the people at this table are from our service, Metro-EMS. Ernie is to my left, barely fitting his legs under the table. His chair is pushed back about two feet farther than mine because his stomach is already butting up against the table.

Tim, my old shell-shocked, douche bag, partner is on my right, staring at somebody across the room that he swears is a sniper. Seriously, Tim is two winks away from a straight-jacket. He's *one* loud noise away from being a slobbering psychology experiment. He'll lose his name and be given a number and that will be that. They'll cart him off to the Stephens Unit. That's where the Thorazine drip comes in. And once they give you that first shot, that's it. You're done. And I know that's Tim's future.

My supervisor—Don (Medic-23)—is beside Tim. Beside Ernie is the Metro-EMS director, Rick, with his wife Samantha. Yes, that's the same hot Samantha that I trained with when I first came to work. She's still hot, and Rick is still chubby and squinty and talks way too fast. Oh, and I think she's sleeping around. Unfortunately, not with me. My suspicions are, to this point, unfounded. But I have one of those intuitive hunches that comes with working around people for long enough to know when their trying to pull a fast one.

My dad always used to tell me not to dip my pen in the company ink. Don says it another way, "Don't put your dick in the cash register."

Either way, they're both correct. It's probably best, especially in this line of work, not to develop personal relationships that might lead to something physical with people you work just inches from. To say it's frowned upon is putting it mildly. But then, almost everyone is doing it, so you just have to be really careful.

Anyway, when we first arrived, they were serving drinks and we were all just mingling, meeting people, stoking up old acquaintances. I ran into these two ER nurses that I had met several times at St. John's Hospital.

Megan and Heather.

Megan had dark brown hair, big brown eyes and perfectly tanned skin that looked fresh out of an electric tanning bed. Heather had short blond hair and deep blue eyes, with thin perfect lips. They were both quite attractive, and I had been waiting for a chance to get either of them alone for quite some time.

Anyway, ever since I talked to them earlier I've been trying to figure out how to approach them. I'm timing my visits to the bar in the back with theirs. About every 17 minutes we meet, I grab a *Jack & Coke*, and they're grabbing glasses of *White Zinfandel*.

We've met about four times now, and I'm thinking this is going to work out in my favor. I excuse myself from the table, barely escaping the gravity that Ernie exerts, and head to the bar. When I get there, Megan and Heather are talking to a guy I've met a few times, named Thomas.

Thomas works for Willard County Ambulance Service. And see, Willard County Ambulance and my company, Metro-EMS, we're basically involved in a turf war, right now. So, this is the paramedic equivalent of a *Crip* and a *Blood* meeting on neutral territory. I kind of nod to Thomas, he kind of nods back. I think I could take him in a fight, not that it would ever come to that. But seriously, I could take him.

Megan takes a sip of wine, "Do you two know each other?"

We both nod again, Megan rolling her eyes. *Boys.*

Heather smiles, approaching me with this sinister sparkle in her eyes. I haven't seen this side of her. Although, usually she's covered in somebody else's blood, so that would obviously cloud over any eye sparkling.

Heather licks her lips, "This is soooo boring."

"I wish we could take this party somewhere else. Turn it up a notch," Megan says. And it's crazy how well girls can read my mind, because I was thinking the same thing.

But where?

"Hey," Thomas says, stepping forward as he lowers his voice, "you know . . . I've got a hot tub at my place. It's not far from here."

I look at Megan, who glances at Heather, who winks at me, who turns and nods to Thomas. "That's a good idea, Thomas. The best idea I've ever heard, tonight."

15 minutes later . . .

I don't know what Thomas was wearing, but I was in my birthday suit. The hot tub was on his back porch, and it was completely dark other than the light from the night's sky. Heather and Megan are wearing their bras and panties, and the wonderful thing is that hot water and alcohol seem to make those garments nearly see-through.

So this is just wonderful by every account. I'm pretty sure I'm getting laid. What I am not so certain about is if it will be with Megan, or with Heather. Megan has been whispering all kinds of filthy things to me all night, so I think she's good to go. But then, Heather has been giving me the eye wink and the tongue on the lips thing, so I might have a shot there, too.

What to do? What to do?

We smoked a little weed in the hot tub, and that seemed to push things along to the next level. Funny how weed will do that very thing. Right now I'm high as a kite, and hard as rock. The girls are primed for action. I can see erect nipples and tongues slowly gliding around mouths that are wanting of pleasure. This is the perfect environment for a life-changing event.

I decided to get things going. Megan slithers over to my right, starting to kiss my neck. Well, decision made. As she starts to kiss me I turn toward her, but I feel something strange. There are three hands on me. Wait . . . maybe four?

I suddenly notice Heather on my left. And her hands that I can't see, are all over my body. This is like what might happen at a physical if it was being performed by porn stars.

I think Thomas must have gotten up to get some drinks or something because I lost track of him. And pretty soon it was a full on three-some! I'm on top of Megan, while Heather is kissing me, water splashing around, fluids being spread in every direction.

Those girls and I did things that would earn a Christian a permanent residence next to Satan's throne. Those ER nurses, for all the horrible, traumatic things they deal with on an everyday basis, they're just full of sexual energy and deviousness.

This will go down as one of the greater feats I had ever accomplished. And then, taken with the fact that it was in enemy territory, in front of a sworn foe . . . it was sheer gold. Well, pink, really, but you get the idea. And, come to think of it, Thomas never said another word to me. Ever.

The score was officially one to nothing. Well, two to nothing if you count the fact that I pissed in the water before leaving.

8
MUTUALLY-ASSURED DESTRUCTION

November 19th
Saturday, 7:08 pm . . .

"Springfield Dispatch to available medical units . . . car pedestrian accident. Thirty-forth and Range Line."

Ernie and I had just sat down at a Krispy Kreme. I was in desperate need of coffee that was strong enough to nurse a hangover. Ernie's trying to gain weight, says it's his '*bulk*' phase or something. So I'm here for coffee, he's here for obesity.

I responded almost immediately, "Metro-three en route!"

A few seconds later we hear, " . . . *Willard County unit-fifteen en route.*"

Ernie and I drop our coffee and donuts. Those bastards are trying to *jump* our call. We run to the unit, start it up, lights and sirens blazing!

Thirty-forth and Range Line is just about 10 or 11 blocks away. So we have to make up time here, or we'll be beat. Again. Willard County unit-15 has been jumping—*stealing*—our calls all week. We can't lose another. It would be too damaging to our morale.

I make sure that I'm behind the wheel for politics' sake. See, Ernie's Benedict Arnold-ass has been working part time at Willard County to support his new wife and inherited kids. Just talking about it makes me mad—his moonlighting, not the kids. He came to work this morning wearing one of their uniforms.

The nerve!

The reason we're involved in this turf war with Willard County is simple: They're a tax-based service. County taxes fund their payrolls. That doesn't leave them with the necessary monies needed to pay for a full-time staff. And trust me, paramedics are 24-7. You always have at least six people, at the bare minimum, on the clock.

So, to offset this deficit in funding and supplement their income they have gone to taking calls in our service area. And that is a big, fat no-no! That's like stomping on toes with a pair of lead boots.

That is the reason I'm breaking all kinds of land-speed records right now. It isn't because of the money. It's because of the principle. Those are our patients. Willard County needs to keep their asses in their own service area!

I race up to about 95 miles an hour, then skid my way back down to just under 10 miles an hour as I California-roll through the stoplights. No sense getting into an accident on the way to an emergency. 95, brake to 10, gas it to 95, brake back to 10—

" . . . *Willard County unit-fifteen is on the scene,*" screeches over the radio.

My knuckles are white. "Son of a bitch!" I barked as I floored it.

"They did it, again!" Ernie says, surprised. Like he's not in on it. Just some innocent bystander. I'm on to him.

As I'm burning through my seventh red light, I say, "Hey, Ernie, didn't you work with Willard County-fifteen last night?"

Avoiding the question, Ernie says, "I'll get the Trauma pack!"

We arrive on the scene moments later. One of the officers controlling the traffic talks to me through the window, "Car-pedestrian. He got his head split open. He's in a *bad* way." And then he looks at me funny, "Hey, how many ambulances are you going to need to transport this guy?"

I scowl at the cop, briefly glancing over at Ernie, "Just one, officer. Just one."

We get out of the unit and jog over to the patient. He's laying in the middle of the brown pavement. And the story is this. The guy was getting piss drunk at a wedding in a hotel on this side of the road. He then decided to walk across the street, in heavy traffic, to where the reception was being held. He found himself going too fast down the hill with no sidewalk for traction.

Being drunk he had limited control over his body and started to lose control. He couldn't stop, and ended up running awkwardly out into the road where a car met his head at 45 miles per hour.

I kneel down. The patient is wearing a light grey shirt, black slacks, a snake skin belt, and a giant gushing head wound.

So we're dealing with another load-and-go, Priority-1 trauma. We can't dick around at this scene. This guy needs an emergency room, *now!*

Ernie, being the consummate non-partisan diplomat, takes over as the experienced medic. He's probably got more than five years of experience on these Willard County guys. All they've really done so far is to maintain in-line stabilization and try to stop some of the bleeding. Ernie does what he does best which is *keeping people alive*. They defer to him instantly.

Meanwhile, I grab a backboard and a gurney so that we can package-up the patient. And in the confusion, the Willard County guys didn't notice as they loaded the patient onto the backboard. They had finished strapping him in before realizing that it was, in fact, *ours*.

By the time they figured out what I had done, we already had the patient rolling toward our ambulance.

"Wait, wait, wait!" one of them yelled as they ran up to us on our way across the grass to the unit. "What are you doing . . . with the patient?"

Ernie kept pushing the cot with the assistance of several firemen as I turned around to face the two bewildered Willard County paramedics. They're standing there, mouths hanging open, their bloody gloves and shirts looking like they just came back from the front lines. Behind me the patient is disappearing into the back of our ambulance.

Ever so slowly, and with as much of a presentation as I could muster, I lifted the radio to just below my mouth, "Metro-three to Springfield Dispatch . . . transporting one to Medical Control. We'll be running hot!"

Running hot means that we're running emergency, and probably going to burn through a bunch of stop lights. *Transporting one* means that we just snatched back our patient. Call it a bamboozle.

As I lower the radio to my hip the guys from Willard County are lowering their heads. This right here, it's priceless. This is the sweet nectar of victory.

I clear my throat and say, "Thanks for holding in-line stabilization for us, fellas." And then I turn and run to the unit that is about to take-off!

Ernie never does say anything about my petty swashbuckling as I jump in the back of the unit. He knows I'm right. And he's about as opinionated as a wind-vane, anyway. Ernie's just happy to be working on a trauma patient who's bleeding profusely. For a guy like him, this is as good as it gets.

A fireman at the wheel, we light 'em up and take off! Ernie and I are working in the back. Victory is coursing through my veins, mixing with the adrenaline of the moment.

I love my job.

You have to understand, for a paramedic, it's all about the trauma call. Not because somebody is going to make a bunch of money. Hell, we get paid by the hour, and not much at that. No, what we're doing is changing the course of life on this planet.

Take this patient for example. Evolution—in the combination of an open bar, a steep hill, and a busy cross street—chose for this man to be taken out of the equation. He was finished.

But here we are, fighting back against the laws of nature, actually making a difference. See, paramedics, different from any other type of medical practitioners, actually affect the immediate outcome of life and death. Go to a hospital and what you have is extended care and medication and all kinds of treatments. But that's just prolonging death. Stringing the grim reaper along.

Trauma is different. Trauma patients will either live or die in my hands. In the back of a dark, bumpy ambulance, traveling at 120 miles an hour. That is raw, undiluted power.

God doesn't save trauma patients . . . we do.

9
THE GREAT TRAIN RACE

December 1th
Thursday, 5:13 pm . . .

"Rural Fire to Springfield Dispatch . . . we have a code blue at the Junction High School gymnasium. Please dispatch a medical unit."

Ernie and I happened to be close to the high school at the moment, and we know we're the only available unit. We had been at Ernie's house where he was showing me his new shotgun. We got in to a discussion of why he needed a gun like that to shoot at squirrels. He didn't have any kind of answer that would hold up in court.

In the middle of our conversation this English Bulldog waddles in, and I just start laughing.

"What's funny?" he had said to me.

The dog is fat and pudgy, and it looks exactly like Ernie. If Ernie got down on all fours and crawled around I'd have a hard time picking one from the other.

I know for a fact that we're the only unit available to respond to the call. All the other Metro-EMS units are transporting patients or answering calls, so I pick up the radio.

"Metro-EMS to Springfield Dispatch . . . Metro-three copies direct. We'll be responding to that call. Please put on standby." And off we go.

Ernie gets behind the wheel and we haul ass. The radio's are alive and excited with all sort of radio traffic from all directions.

As we approach the school, one of the first responders—volunteers—comes over the radio, saying, *"Metro unit responding . . . we have a twelve-year-old cardiac arrest here at the basketball game. Bystanders started CPR. We're continuing it."*

I grab the radio immediately, "Metro-three to Life-Flight, please be en route. We'll set-up an LZ (landing zone) outside Junction High School."

"LifeFlight copy."

Both luck and fate seemed to be conspiring against us as we neared the school. Here's the problem. There are only two access points to this area, where the high school is located. Both of the entrances are separated by no less than five miles. There's no in-between.

And looking at this entrance road, we see a train bearing down on us, about to cross our road. And it's one of those long 15-minute trains that seem to last forever. The crossing gates have already lowered across the road, all kinds of blinking red lights and obnoxious bells are sounding.

And we're on a real clock, here. This kid is in cardiac arrest. Brain death occurs in 4-6 minutes. So if we make a 10-mile detour—five to the other entrance, and five back to the school—this kid will be either a permanent vegetable, or outright dead.

We're about a quarter of a mile away from the crossing, pedal to the metal, closing in on it at an intense velocity. Ernie asks, "What do you think, Danny? Detour, or . . ." and then he glances at the tracks where the train is quickly approaching.

"It's a twelve-year-old, Ernie," I remind him.

He nods, tightening his grip on the steering wheel, lowering his huge shoulders, "Hold on, then!"

I make the sign of the cross and prepare for a collision.

Ernie, using a rare blend of skill and luck, manages to thread the gates at a ridiculous rate of speed, with the train honking its ear-shattering air horn at us. We are so damn close that we actually felt the thick cushion of air in the front of the train pushing us away from the tracks as we raced by.

If there had been contact, it would have been incredibly grisly. We would have exploded like a space shuttle. It would take CSI to find all of our bits and pieces.

One minute and forty-eight seconds later we are skidding to a stop in the Junction High School parking lot. We grab the *Lifepack-10*, Airway bag, drug box, and follow the first responders into the gymnasium where probably a thousand people are watching all of this unfold. The stadium was packed, every seat filled, but it was eerily quiet.

For most of these kids, this is the first time they've watched somebody they know die right in front of them.

Luckily for the kid, the woman doing the CPR was a nurse, so she was doing it properly. We take over the patient and I begin to intubate as the nurse explains what happened.

The 12-year-old in front of us fell like a sack of potatoes during a basketball game. People thought he had just tripped, but when he didn't get up, people realized something else was wrong. Turns out he has a congenital heart defect.

He's pale and clammy, with the color completely drained from his body. He's wearing his yellow and blue uniform, and looks more like a mannequin than a human child. And I know he doesn't have much time.

Ernie slaps the *fast-patches*—hand-sized defibrillator pads that are ultra sticky and incredibly conductive—on the boy's lower left chest, and upper right chest. In the 1960s people used those paddles you see on television all the time, but they don't get near the conduction. Also, the fast-patches are hooked-up to the monitor. That gives us all kinds of important information about the patient's heart.

So, when we're trying to jump-start somebody's heart, we use the fast-patches.

By the time I get the intubation done, Ernie is yelling, "He's in v-fib, everyone clear!" Think *quivering, uncoordinated* heart.

We all pull our hands up and he shocks the patient. The boy's chest lifts off the floor as his muscles contract from the surge of electricity, and then back down to the hardwood floor.

I let a fireman breathe for him using a BVM while I start an IV. Meanwhile, Ernie's assessing the cardiac rhythm. Another fireman is doing the chest compressions.

And no sooner do I get the IV started that Ernie yells, "Everyone clear!"

We all pull our hands up, zap! The patient lifts, drops, and we're back at it.

The fireman resumes breathing and chest compressions while I administer a bolus—large amount, dosage —of epinephrine. And by the time the plunger is pressing against the plastic, Ernie is ready to shock the patient again.

"Everyone clear!" he says, sweating and breathing hard. I'm really hoping that Ernie doesn't fall over next to this kid clutching *his* heart. Because I'll be in deep brown stuff then.

Everything we're doing, Ernie and me and the firemen, it's like a smoothly orchestrated cascade of events. It's as if we've practiced together a thousand times for this one moment. But really we've learned from the dead and dying in our past. The ghosts in the back of our minds taught us what we now do as a matter of reaction.

Ernie shocks the boy a third time, and just as the firemen goes to start the chest compressions again, he yells, "Hold on, he's got a rhythm! Check his pulse."

I check the carotid artery on his neck and find a pulse. We then continue using the BVM to breathe for him. The fireman squeezes his hand, sending a fresh breath of 100% pure oxygen into the boy's lungs.

I give him a shot of lidocaine to stabilize his cardiac rhythm, and we package him up carefully. We place him on the backboard, setting the oxygen bottle between his legs. Ernie throws the monitor over his shoulder by its strap so that he can continue to read the patient's vital signs.

The boy is starting to look better with every passing second. He's gaining color, looking less plastic and deathly. We lift him onto the gurney and head toward the gym door. And the moment we get there, the double doors being held open, I see the LifeFlight helicopter parked so close it's almost surreal. It doesn't look like it belongs here.

We race across the short stretch of parking lot and load him into the helicopter while I explain to the flight nurse all of the pertinent information. And before we know it the helicopter is taking off with the boy.

Seconds later they disappear into the darkening clouded sky, the rumble of the propeller fading quickly. And then . . . they're gone. Vanished. It's like none of it ever happened.

And you know what, that Goddamn train still hasn't passed us, yet. Ernie and I gather up our gear and head out to our unit.

"Good job beating that train, Ernie," I tell him, giving him a slap on the shoulder. "You saved that kid."

He nodded, "*We* did, Danny. We did."

That Ernie, he makes you want to be a better human. He's so good-hearted that I want to call up ex-girlfriends and apologize for stuff I never even did. He gives me a glimpse of what decency really is. I like my big, fat, donut-guzzling, virgin partner.

I could tell you about the time he was cleaning one of his pistols and accidentally shot a hole in the center of his giant hand. I mean it was right through the dead center of his palm. You could look right through the hole, it was that big. And, luckily for him, it seemed to miss every bone and major vein and tendon. None of us could believe that he wasn't badly hurt. We had no problem with the fact that he shot himself. That was almost a given. As if, when he purchased the gun it came with a special warning just for Ernie about what he should do when he shot himself.

But all of that, it doesn't do anything to take away from how decent a person Ernie really is. His level of compassion is bigger than he and his portly bulldog put together. And there's nobody I'd rather have picking me up off the pavement.

10
STUMPED

May 5th
Friday, 6:43 pm . . .

"Springfield Dispatch to Metro-EMS . . . we have a man found on the side of Fountain Road. Caller states that the man is requesting help and is covered in blood."

Ernie and I are walking down the middle of a Walmart, looking for supplies for a dinner we're going to cook back at the station. We're at an impasse because he wants to get regular ground beef, but I want ground chuck—the good stuff. We already have a cart full of food, just ready to go. We have vegetables, buns, soda, barbecue sauce. And the butcher is waiting for our argument to stop so that he can give us our meat.

Looking across the cart at each other, neither of us speaks. We're waiting to see if anyone else is going to answer this call. We've spent the last 45 minutes shopping, filling up this cart, and if we have to go now, we'll never eat. The night is going to be ruined, for sure.

Breaking the silence we hear our supervisor, Don, respond, *"Metro-EMS to Springfield Dispatch . . . "*

And then we hold our breath.

" . . . *Metro-three will be responding.*"

Damn it!

We back away from the cart, maybe a little slower than we should have. "Come on, Ernie . . . they'll be other meals."

We turn and jog, Ernie talking under his breath. We don't run. As a matter of fact, we *never* run, especially at a scene. You see, running at a scene causes panic. And panic spreads like wildfire. Maybe not in a Walmart, but we still don't run.

"Medic-twenty-three, this is Medic-thirteen . . . we copy that. We're en route from Walmart," I say as we make our way out of the store.

We hop in the unit, light 'em up and head out.

As we begin our race to the patient we start to hear first responders on the scene describing what they believe happened. From what we're hearing, it's a bloody nightmare. There's some guy, no vehicle in sight. He's got blood and mud all over him. He's incoherent, not responding well.

Ernie is psyched about this. He's rubbing the belly of the Trauma buddha, thanking him for such a wonderful gift. Because, the more these guys talk on the radio, the more horrible it all sounds.

Because it's so far out, it takes us a relatively long time to get to the scene. When we finally arrive there are half a dozen first responders. They've started to bandage up the guy. There is just blood everywhere. Everybody's rubber gloves are wet sticky red.

We're thinking that this is a murder. Maybe somebody dropped him out of a car, or out of a plane. Something impossibly frightening. The kind of stuff urban legends are made of.

One of the early responders meet us as we're getting out of the vehicle. "The guy says he's from town and he came out here for work. Says there was an accident on the job site."

As we approached we could smell the ammonia and the familiar spoiled milk smell that *is* Billy Angel. Both Ernie and I groan and sigh at the same time.

As soon as he sees us, Billy says, "There's no need to have the fucking cops here. We don't need no cops."

"We're not cops, Billy. We're paramedics," I say. The guy still doesn't recognize us. I see the sorry bastard every shift and he treats each meeting like it's our first.

As Ernie is cutting away at his blood-soaked pants, I start asking questions. "What did you do to yourself, Billy?"

To which he replies, "I didn't do nuthin'. And it's none of your business, anyway. Just fix my leg, cop."

"We're paramedics, Billy."

"Fix . . . my . . . leg . . . pig!"

It's obvious he's lost a significant amount of blood and he's going to need to go the hospital. He's acting loopier than normal.

Ernie looks up at me, "There's splinters of wood sticking out of his leg."

"There's one in my ass, too," Billy adds. "And it hurts."

We go about the business of packing him up. We give him the full trauma immobilization—C-collar, towel rolls, backboard, dressings over the gaping wounds. We start an IV because he's definitely going to need blood when he gets to the hospital.

We thank the volunteers as we're loading him up into the unit, congratulating them on a job well done. Since they don't get paid, a *thank you* from a paramedic is a nice enough reward. They get to be part-time heroes, and they do save lives. Without them our jobs would be considerably more difficult.

This is a Priority-2, so I'm driving while Ernie tends to Billy in the back of the unit. I instantly roll the windows down because he smells so incredibly bad. The kind of wretched odor that makes you gag.

I yell back, "Ernie, see if you can find out what happened to him."

You see, if he was assaulted we *have* to call the police. It becomes a criminal matter. But as it turns out, that's not at all the case.

After a muffled discussion, Ernie gives me the short of it, "He says he was blowin' stumps!"

By *blowin' stumps* he means to say, using high-order explosives to remove tree stumps from the ground. This is a dangerous and technical skill, to be practiced only by licensed professionals. Unless you're from our town. Then you find the most expendable person you can, and con him into doing it for drinking money.

During the long ride to the hospital, Ernie communicates with Billy. He has good bedside manner. He's much more considerate and understanding of our patient's emotional needs than I am. For me it's a business. For Ernie, there's much more to it. There's a human component. He cares.

And so he precedes to establish rapport with Billy as we drive. In the back I can hear them talking while Ernie continues to stave off the bleeding.

And here's what we learn along the way: Apparently, a tree-removal service had gotten a contract to clear a plot of land outside of town. They have machines that turn tree stumps into saw dust that are used for the majority of the clearing process. However, they occasionally run into trees that are too large for the machine. In those instances, they are forced to use explosives to uproot the stumps.

There was a group of particularly nasty tree stumps that they realized would be a dangerous affair to remove. Obviously, using explosives in the middle of nowhere is a dangerous undertaking. That's when one of the contractors had the bright idea to hire some homeless guy to do the dirty work.

Billy Angel is a lot of things, but he's no explosives expert. I'm not sure what kind of on-the-job training you get for blowing trees up, but it apparently wasn't sufficient. When you mix Billy and dynamite, you just can't have a happy ending. Really, when you mix Billy and just about anything it gets ugly.

But especially explosives.

What seems to have occurred is that he wasn't at the minimum safe distance away from one of the stumps when he initiated the explosive charge. Jagged shards of the stump embedded themselves deep into his legs, arms, chest, and ass.

Yes . . . his *ass*.

The scary thing is, looking at his injuries, he must have done it more than once. That's the only way to explain all the injuries. Billy's got drive, I'll give him that. When he says he's going to do something, even if it will surely kill him, he'll do it.

I grab the radio, "Metro-three to Medical control . . . we're inbound with a Priority-two trauma patient."

And I don't want to tell them who this patient happens to be, but I have to, " . . . it's Billy Angel."

I don't hear anything for an awkward pregnant pause. And then, after a few seconds of static and barely audible sighing, I hear, *"Copy that Metro-three . . . we'll have his room ready."*

I realize that I probably ruined a bunch of people's night with that call, but I had to give them fair warning.

The Angel is coming.

11
FREIGHT TRAINING

July 29th
Saturday, 2:17 pm . . .

My pager starts screaming like a banshee! I lift myself up off the couch and reach for the wooden end table where my pager is shuffling around. I scoop it up and glance at the small screen,

'On call . . . report to station!'

There goes my easy Friday. See, we get five on-call days per month. Usually it means that if there's a serious emergency we'll be called in to man the station while everyone else heads out in the units.

But not this time.

Not this call.

I slipped on my boots, flipped off the television, and jumped into my Ford Ranger. On a good day I can make it to the station from my apartment in just under 12 minutes. On a bad day, if the traffic is ugly, it might take me 25.

Today wasn't a good day, but I still made it in 13 minutes. That should have been my first clue. The initial foreshadowing of what I was going to be dealing with. But you don't think like that. At least, I don't. No, 13 minutes is just four songs and a commercial. Just a stretch of lights and music.

I made my way into the station and it was a ghost town. Everybody was out on calls. My on-call partner walked in about 30 seconds behind me.

Samantha—the hot chick paramedic, and the director's wife—was going to be sitting in the station with me for the next few hours. Normally this is the point where we grab a soda, kick back and relax, maybe get some paperwork done.

But that wasn't the case.

Over the radio we kept hearing, *"**Metro-one . . . please advise if you're at the station, yet.**"*

Metro-one is the call-sign for the station. That means, Metro-one is us—Samantha and me. We look at each other, knowing that we are going to have to go out on this one. Whatever it is, they don't have enough help on the scene.

"Metro-one copies . . . on-call is at the station," Samantha responds.

*"**Metro-one . . . procede to north Main at the train trussel. Respond immediately!**"*

We race to the garage and jump into one of the units. Samantha is driving, I'm riding shotgun. She picks up the radio, "Metro unit-five en route."

Six minutes later we find ourselves pulling onto an abandoned road, mostly covered in grass and small brush. About a 100 yards down the path we see tons of emergency vehicles. There are two ambulances, three police cars, and a firetruck, already on scene.

There's an adult male, sitting on the ground, his knees pulled up to his chest. His head is down and he's sobbing uncontrollably. Two police officers are near him, not really asking questions, just talking quietly.

We fast walk past him and he doesn't even look up. This scene is disconcertingly quiet. Nobody is talking. There's no yelling. Everyone is just solemnly walking back and forth.

The firemen wave us up to the top of the trussel. And I remember this place. Occasionally people will come out here to jump off of the trussel into the water down below. It's only about 15 feet high. Just enough to get your heart racing, but low enough that you're not going to die if you do a belly-flop. You know, just a couple hours of summer fun.

On our way up a fireman walks by, his eyes hollow and vacant as if he's seen something that he's not supposed to be able to see. He's witnessed something we're not designed for. And in a barely audible voice he says, "That's it . . . I'm done. That's fuckin' it."

The problem with this location is that you have to jump from the train tracks that run across the top. There isn't a lot of room up here on either side of the tracks.

We make our way up to the top of the trussel and we see blood and bits of bone and hair, *everywhere*. There are several body bags already. Two medics, assisted by several firemen, are working on a small child, who's missing his left arm.

"We can't find his arm," one of the firefighters said, his face rather flush, his brow moist with sweat. "It's got to be around here. It just has to."

The child was right beside the tracks, completely pale. Totally unresponsive; which, under the circumstances was probably good. They were getting him packaged-up when we got there.

Not more then five feet away were the remains of a 4-year-old that had been chopped in half at the lower abdomen. The other bodies were even less put together. The firefighters were collecting tiny parts in different bags, trying to match the size of the arms and legs, with the torsos that were left.

And there isn't much to work with. If I was to guess, I'd say there might be three different children, chopped into almost unrecognizable, stomach-turning pieces. And they were all DRTs.

Dead right there.

Samantha and I were instantly tasked with taking the small boy to the hospital before he bled out. And time was short for him. There was so much to see, and it was all so horrible, that my mind couldn't compute it.

It didn't make any sense.

This is probably why most paramedics suffer the long term effects of post-traumatic stress disorder.

What was explained to us by the fireman that drove our ambulance was this: The family of six—the stepfather that we had passed, and his five young children —had been taking turns jumping off of the train trussel into the water. Just having a relaxing summer afternoon together. The tracks that lead to the trussel take a sharp turn less than a hundred meters away, behind a thick mat of trees. Basically, the train had come out of nowhere when four of the five kids had been up on the trussel preparing to jump.

As the train rounded the corner the children were taken by surprise. Kids don't stand much chance against a freight train. Three of the children—two girls and a boy, all under the age of 10—were smashed to pieces before they could even react.

The fourth child, that we were transporting, had only caught the edge of the train, tore his arm off halfway up the humerus. And he was leaking badly.

The only two to remain unharmed were the step-dad and one of the girls, who had just jumped into the water seconds earlier. Chances are, she was smiling and laughing, splashing down into the water while her brothers and sisters were being decimated.

The step-dad, he got to watch it all happen. Every gory second. Most likely, he's finished. And not from a legal standpoint, but from a psychological one. With that kind of thing, and the amount of guilt and personal responsibility that comes with it, there's no way he'll ever be a full person again. That magnitude of tragedy, especially if you have any culpability—both real or imagined—spins your mind in directions that all the pharmaceuticals in the world can't fix.

People can say what they want to comfort him. But he'll know *he* killed them. Sure it was a train that came out of nowhere. Yes, people have been jumping off of the train trussel for 50 years. I'm sure he was a great dad.

But still, he killed them. That's all he'll ever remember.

We used a thick trauma dressing to cover the entire arm of the young boy in order to stave off the blood loss, and my lunch. We got him to the unit, and to the hospital in minutes.

When we finally delivered the child to the ER, Samantha looked at me, breathing deeply. She needed to get away from this. We drove to an empty parking lot where I left her alone in the cab while I went out and smoked a cigarette.

I'd been smoking a lot, lately. Maybe drinking a little more than I should have been, too. You can't help it. Something *has* to take the edge off. Or you'll just pop. Life in full color is too much. Especially when the color is red.

I was leaning against the back of the ambulance, smoking to calm my nerves. Puffing away at poison and nicotine so that I wouldn't have to think about what I'd just been a part of. She was in the cab, sobbing because she *was* thinking about it.

She and I, we'll both eventually end up at the same place. We're just starting from different locations. This life of ours is a crooked line. I'm going to sit out here and smoke until somebody tells me otherwise . . . or I run out of cigarettes. Because, I don't have the money for a good shrink.

Everything that you do as a paramedic to forget the horrible events we get to routinely experience, I'm pretty certain they're the exact opposite of what are considered *healthy* psychological coping skills. At some point, you just stop looking at your fingernails because there's so much dried blood underneath them.

Burnout . . . I figure that's when you look down at your fingers and you can't see the blood at all. I'm not there, yet.

The immediate effect of this was emotional wreckage. Everyone was damaged. We had a CISD (Critical Incident Stress Debriefing). That's where all of the emergency workers can meet up and discuss what happened. There are all of these psychologists and other mental health professionals to help guys deal with post-traumatic stress, and any of the other kinds of emotional scarring.

This particular CISD was hosted at St. John's, and I remember it distinctly because so many people broke down. It was like some kind of freaking nightmare. Lots of people quit working over that. Seasoned fire-fighters, nurses, paramedics, and even a doctor. Like that firefighter that had passed us on the way to the tressel. . .

. . . they were *done*.

12
A PERFECT ANGEL

October 12th
Saturday night...

"Springfield Dispatch to Metro-EMS . . . medical call, sexual assault. Ninth and Main, in the alley."

I lift my radio, "Metro-three en route. Please have officers respond." I lower the radio to my side, nodding to Ernie. We just finished cleaning the unit, so we were only two feet away. I didn't even have my radio back on my hip when I was shutting the passenger door.

Ernie lit 'em up, hit the sirens, and we squealed out of the bay on our way to the call. And we're there almost instantly because it's only a couple of blocks from the station.

When we get there the police are on the scene, and one of the officers waves me over to warn, "Just so you know . . . it's Billy Angel."

We walk around to discover our dear friend Mr. Angel laying on his back in the alley. He looks as old and disgusting as ever, but with an added bonus. His musty old pants are down to his ankles. As we approach I notice a new bottle of *Wild Turkey* in his left hand. His right hand is balled into an angry fist. He looks madder than a sack full of cats.

The first thing I say to him is, "Damn it, Billy . . . I spend more time with you than I do my own family."

"Fuck you, you . . . you don't know what I go through. It's horrible! Keep those faggots off of me. Did you catch them?"

Catch *who*, Billy?

He sits halfway up, "The queers, man! Did you catch the queers, yet? Look what they done."

"Slow down, Billy," I said. "Just take a breath and relax."

Nobody, no matter who they are, should have to be sexually abused. Rape isn't funny, even if Billy occasionally is. The strong aren't supposed to prey on the weak. This is the uglier side of humanity. The side of life that nobody should ever have to witness.

I glance over at Ernie and his eyes are almost watering. He's taking this differently than I am. Ernie's kind of an empath. What we try and do now is retain what dignity Billy has left.

And I'll be honest, I actually feel pretty bad for this guy. We cover him in a thick blanket, carefully load him onto the cot and take him to the unit. In the kindest gesture I've ever made, I go back and gather up all of his trash and belongings, throwing them in the back of the unit.

I tell the officers to follow us to the hospital so that they can make an official report and a rape kit—semen samples, finger prints, DNA. The whole nine yards. Billy's body is a crime scene until the investigation is complete. This is why it's so important to get rape victims to the hospital as quickly as possible. Evidence starts to disappear almost from the second of the crime. If you wait hours, it might be too late.

I wish . . . I wish that just once I could help this guy. For good. I wish there was a way to give this guy a shot and inoculate him against all the pain and suffering he must feel on a daily basis. In the cold space of the universe, there is no morality. No right and wrong, or fair and unfair. But here, in the unforgiving streets that we all take for granted, guys like Billy are victimized by the rest of us. Like it or not, we made him.

He's our dad.

Our brother.

Our kid.

When I go to take his pulse, at his wrist, I notice his clenched hand again. "Billy . . . what's in your hand?"

He kind of shrugs and looks away. But he won't open his hand.

"I need to check your pulse, so you need to relax your hand."

I can see the tendons tightening down on the underside of his wrist.

"Billy," I order him, "open your hand, now!"

He glares at me, his eyes just two little slits.

I sigh, "Billy, please open your hand. It's alright. I'm not going to hurt you. I need to take your pulse."

He snorts through his nose, and shakes his head. Slowly his hand opens up to reveal two crinkled 50-dollar bills.

Oh, *crap*. I close my eyes, looking up to the ambulance's ceiling. I should have seen this coming. You allow yourself an ounce of emotional investment, and you get cheated quicker than a Vegas slot machine.

I shake my head sadly, "You didn't get raped, did you?"

He opens his mouth to reply, but all that comes out is a half breath, barely enough to be audible.

I turn my head up, yelling toward the front of the unit, "Save your tears, Ernie. This one's a *workin'* girl!"

But Ernie is such a virgin, completely inept when it comes to things like this, that he doesn't understand what I'm talking about. "Huh?" he replies.

"He was whoring himself out," I explain. "Our man is a man-whore."

And then I look down at Billy, "So . . . you care to explain this before the cops start asking you questions you can't possibly answer?"

"I needed the money, man," he says. "Everything was fine until the guy pulls out somethin' meant to split me into two pieces."

I'm noticeably cringing, trying to delete any imagery relating to Billy Angel having violent gay sex for money. So I try and change the subject, "Hey, uh, I notice you're healing-up pretty well from the stump blowing incident."

He nods, "Yeah, they took the cast off last week. Still got the staples, though. That dynamite is a bitch, huh!" And then the weirdest smile makes his face crooked for a moment. Then it's gone.

I look down at his staples, "Those look kind of rusted."

"Yeah, they were supposed to take them out a while ago. Couple weeks, I think."

Billy absolutely cannot take care of himself. Every day he wakes up is another middle finger at evolution. He's continually taunting fate. Each step he takes, somewhere a statistic is being rewritten.

I guess I should have expected each and every part of this God-awful story.

I pick up my radio, taking in a deep breath and groaning, "Metro-three to Medical control . . . we have a fifty-year-old sexual assault. Patient is stable and in a comfortable position. We'll be at your facility in five minutes."

We take him to the hospital and deliver him to the emergency room staff. Recognizing him instantly, they then direct us to Billy's *usual* room. Ernie and I go to rid the ambulance of all smells that remind us of Billy.

After I finish my requisite cigarette, I take his belongings up to his room. At this point I'm just ambling down the hall, wanting to wash my hands and take a shower. I feel dirty. Disgusting. Maybe I need to go to confession at the local church, who knows.

As I get out of the elevator I notice one of the nurses dashing frantically out of his room, her hands covering her mouth, as she cuts a direct path to the employee bathrooms. I go to drop off his stuff in the room and I overhear one of the doctors asking him,

" . . . Billy . . . how long have you had *maggots* in your ass?"

Mr. Angel—since he's in the hospital he's a *Mr.* now —really doesn't have an answer for this question. He's not his usual charismatic self.

The doctor shrugs, turning to me, "Well, they probably kept him clean. They eat the bacteria, you know."

In my entire life I've never felt sorrier for maggots than right now. The horrors they must have suffered living in Billy's ass. It gives me a full-body quiver. I have all sorts of unnerving questions bouncing around in my mind, but I *know* that I won't ever be able to eat again if I get the answers.

I drop the bag full of Billy's trash, turn on my heel, and head out into the hall. A pair of nurses fast-walk by murmuring something about, " . . . had actual live maggots in his . . . "

I'm heading outside, now, where I can have a few more cigarettes. When I finally get to the unit, Ernie is sitting on the back, with the rear doors open, staring numbly at the pavement. He looks distraught, saddened deeply by this. He doesn't get this depressed after a multiple fatality with a chainsaw. But there's something about Billy that really gets to Ernie.

"What's up, Ernie?" I ask delicately.

He slowly lifts his head, his eyes red, "There's just no hope for some people, huh?"

I pull a cigarette out, lighting it with a cheap blue lighter. I take a long, slow drag, and offer one to

Ernie. He lifts his big, meaty arm and takes one. The cigarettes look like match sticks in his huge hands.

I reach over and light it for him and we just sit there, letting our thoughts evaporate with the soft grey smoke as it dissipates above us.

13
DEFENSIVE DRIVING

November 22nd
Wednesday, 9:53 pm . . .

"Springfield Dispatch to Metro-EMS . . . medical call, gastro-intestinal bleed. The caller says the patient is in and out of consciousness. Country Living Nursing Home on North Main and Fountain Road."

I was with my supervisor—Don (*Medic-23*)—and we're both working an extra shift to get some Christmas money. We don't usually get to work together because he's a supervisor and I'm a crew chief, so this is a nice change.

Don picks up the radio, "Metro-four is en route." We had just left his house, picking up some dinner that his wife had cooked for us. It was a lasagna and it smelled absolutely divine.

I'm driving, and we've got the full deal—lights and sirens blaring. The roads are slicked with ice, so I'm only going about 45 or 50 miles per hour. The roads were basically empty, like this was a ghost town.

Typically, when a passenger vehicle sees us coming they will pull to the right and let us pass. Typically.

Well, we come up behind a red Firebird and he pulls slowly to the right, like we would expect. So I start to accelerate past him. But, for reasons that are still far beyond my comprehension, he suddenly turns back to the left, crossing directly in front of us.

And there's no stopping it.

I did everything I could, sliding to the left, but it didn't help. All I did was take out a light pole in the process. So now, an ambulance and a light pole are about to smash him.

We T-bone him in the dead center of his little red car!

After we skidded to a stop, I checked my supervisor to make sure he's alright. See, our ambulance is an older model, and at that time not all ambulances came equipped with airbags. Luckily we had our seatbelts on so we didn't get injured.

"Don," I yelled, "are you alright?!"

He just looked at me, shook his head and said, "Shooooo." Absolutely nothing excites this guy. After so many years of emergency medicine, he's been mined of all his *give-a-shit*. I wonder if the guy even gets erections, anymore.

I jump out of the ambulance to help this kid in the Firebird while Don grabs the radio to check on the status of the other available ambulances.

I'm running with the Trauma pack toward the car and I can hear, " *. . . Metro-five is transporting organ-procurement team.*"

I notice this young kid, maybe 16 or 17, and he's jerking around. What's happening is a trauma-induced seizure. These kinds of seizures happen often, directly after a traumatic accident. Oddly, there is still no medical term for these types of seizures. And you know how doctors like to give long frustrating names to everything.

Not that it matters, I'm still going to treat him using the normal trauma protocols. I take in-line stabilization—controlling the patient's neck—from the driver's side door. It's important to hold the spine right away. Any movement could kill him instantly if he's got a compromised spine. You might not see anything, and then he moves a quarter of an inch and he's dead or paralysed.

Right then.

No warning.

As I'm holding his neck, asking him questions, I hear my radio, " . . . *Metro-six still has neo-natal isolette and staff on board.*"

That's all three ambulances.

Immediately Don's voice comes across the radio, saying, "*Metro-EMS to Springfield Dispatch . . . please call in all on-call staff. Dispatch Willard County Ambulance to our call. Our unit is out-of-service. Please dispatch police and fire to Fifth and Main.*"

They ask for more information and Don explains that we've just been in an accident and that we have on-scene injuries to take care of. This goes on and on while I'm holding this kid's neck.

And here's what is about to happen: Willard County—our competitors-turned-allies—are going to be dispatched to our original call, the female gastro-intestinal bleed at the nursing home. We're not thinking about some silly turf war right now because, ultimately, what is important is keeping people alive.

Our on-call paramedics will be coming to assist us at *this* scene. The one we created.

Don comes over quickly with the backboard and C-collars. We begin to package-up and treat the kid who is no longer seizing. He didn't have any obvious outward signs of injury, and was doing much better.

We get him on a cot and roll him to the back of our unit, which is now completely cluttered with equipment and supplies all over the place. A crash will do that. But we have to put him inside because it's important to keep him warm until the back-up unit arrives.

And it doesn't take long before *everybody* is here! Police cars are pulling up. Firetrucks. Our director, Gary. Pretty much everyone we can imagine. This is a bad thing. I'm thinking that my career is probably over. I crashed an ambulance, into a kid, on the way to a call.

We went from being participants in a collision, directly into paramedic-caregiver mode. And I'm completely drained, almost on the verge of collapse.

Thankfully, Gary pulls me aside and tells me that if I'm not hurt, and after everything is taken care of on the scene, for us to just go on home, and we'll deal with all this in the morning.

Don opted to stay at the accident scene, and I decided to continue patient care. So when the on-call paramedics arrived I went with them and the patient to the hospital. If the doctors had any questions about the accident, or to determine the *mechanism of injury*, then I would be the best person to provide answers.

We have to paint the best possible picture of the accident scene. This is so that doctors know exactly what they're looking for. Hospitals are so disconnected and removed from the actual chaos that it is important to have reliable firsthand knowledge of exactly what occurred.

When we arrived at the hospital, the parents were already there. They see us and like angry dogs they're on me, yelling and accusing me. And at this point, I don't really have an good answers for them. What can I say?

Yes, we hit your kid . . . but it was his fault.

"What did you do to our son?!" the mother screams. "Who the hell do you think you—"

But a doctor comes to my rescue, interrupting their shouting. "Ma'am," he says sternly, "your son turned in front of an ambulance that was running emergency. And you know what . . . a woman is dead now, because *they* couldn't answer that call."

And then everybody got quiet. Now it's not about a wrecked car, or how their precious child was endangered by a reckless paramedic.

After we describe everything about the accident to the doctors, recounting every detail I can recall, I head back to the station to fill out an incident report and give my statement to the police. They require this immediately so I don't forget anything. It's only fresh in your mind one time. Everything after that is patch-work.

Then I got in my little Ford Ranger and drove home. And when I got there I just melted into oblivion, eating my portion of the cold, yet heavenly, lasagna.

By that time in my career I have so much horrible stuff floating around in my head that it is starting to surface at inappropriate times. I might be at a gas station, or in a supermarket, and just the smell of something, or a flash of color, or even the location would bring back a flood of terrible memories. And I couldn't control the barrage of imagery.

I have had to figure out a way to cope. At first it was just a drink or two. A 6-pack, tops. Then I was taking shots. Then I graduated past liquor to smoking weed. I followed the proverbial stair steps up until I was flirting with cocaine on the side.

Nothing I couldn't control, of course.

Just self-medicating.

14
BEAR-HORSE ATTACK!

December 9th
Somewhere in Kansas . . .

So my partner Ernie and I are out in the middle of *Nowhere*, Kansas, doing a non-emergency transfer. We were taking this nice elderly woman back from the hospital to a nursing home. She's all fixed and ready to go back to the home and eat rasin soup, or rice gruel, or whatever the hell it is they feed them.

Out in the middle of nowhere there is absolutely no traffic, no people, no life whatsoever. You pretty much keep the hammer down, making as good time as possible. Ernie is driving, and I'm in the back with the lady, playing *Duke Nuke'em* on my laptop.

I'm gunning down all kinds of zombies that have no business trying to eat me, and every five minutes I check on the patient. Each time I look at her vital signs and make sure she's still comfortable, I've killed another 25 monsters. So, I'm being fairly productive.

Out on the open road Ernie has a rather peculiar tendency to spread his wings and fly. And by fly I mean to haul unholy ass.

I'm unloading a chain-gun on some giant undead dogs and I feel this sudden bump. Now, my back is to the front of the unit, so I hardly even notice. And the lady is firmly locked in place. She's got leg straps, abdominal straps, and chest straps that come over the shoulder. She's not going anywhere.

But, what is particularly odd is that everything is now silent. I don't hear the ambulance's engine noise, the sound of the road, or anything else for that matter. I made sure the patient was alright and then I started to see smoke or something drifting through the air. But it wasn't smoke at all. It was the gas out of one of those fancy new airbag thingies. They leave a thick powder residue.

I turn toward the front, "Hey Ernie, you alright?"

He doesn't answer right away. I guess he was stunned.

"Ernie? What's up, buddy?"

"We . . . we hit a bear."

A what?

"We hit a Black Bear," he answers.

Really loud I said, "Ernie, there's no bears in Kansas. What's the matter with you?"

"Ah, hang on . . . I'm going to check and see what happened."

"Goddammit, Ernie, if it *was* a bear we hit, and we didn't kill it, it's going to be pissed-off! Really pissed-off!"

"Okay," he answered groggily, "I'm going to take that into consideration during my search."

It's obvious that Ernie is punch drunk.

The elderly woman turns her head to me, in the softest, most tender voice she asks, "Did he say we hit a . . . bear?"

"No, sweetie," I answer delicately, "bears don't live in Kansas. There's nothing for them to do here. My partner Ernie just got a little ding on his head. He'll be fine."

"That's nice," she says, closing her eyes.

Ernie gets out, searching for God-only-knows what. The unit still has power so I get on the radio and contact our station. When I explained what had happened their first words were, "Not again!"

I assure them I wasn't the one driving. I hate to throw Ernie under the bus like that, but it is what it is. I ask them send another ambulance, and to have a wrecker start this way.

Ernie opens the back door and sticks his head in, letting out all the heat. By this time I had put my black highway-patrol cap on the patient's head to keep her warm. It has those cool ear flaps to keep you toasty. She was a sight.

He says, "Good news . . . it was only a horse." Then he shrugs, "Open range policy."

"What does that mean?" I ask. Ernie is originally from Kansas, so he's the kind of guy who would know stuff like that.

"It means they let their cattle and farm animals go wherever they'd like," he explains.

"That sounds like the most stupid narrow-sighted policy ever created in the history of history. People come down the highway at seventy and smash into *Black Beauty*, or *Elsie*."

"We were way over seventy," he smiles as he corrects me.

"Whatever, Ernie. You know what I mean."

I have Ernie stay with the patient while I get out and take a look around. There is half of a horse right next to the back of the unit. There is a spray of horse crap all over the driver's side of the unit. And it was liquefied. This is the kind of crap that comes from inside the intestines.

The unit itself was completely inoperable, the entire front end folded impossibly on itself. We weren't going anywhere under our own power. While I was outside assessing the damage I had him call his friends from the closest Kansas ambulance service. Coincidentally, he had actually worked for one of them. They would have to take over patient care and deliver her to the nursing home.

There are long skidded lines of guts and bits and pieces everywhere. It looks like he exploded on impact, but strangely the horse was cleanly severed in half, as if a giant sword had chopped him in two.

In this case, the sword's name was *Ernie*.

We wait for about 30 minutes and then the Kansas paramedics arrive to take over patient care. I give them a briefing on her. They load her into their unit and go. No coffee, or small talk. Just a quick transfer and then off into the blackness of the night. I got the impression they didn't like us.

Ernie and I wait around in the darkness until the Chuck shows up. Not Mr. Chuck, or Chuck. No, it's *the Chuck*. He's one of a kind.

And he's all smiles and giggling as he eyeballs the mess we've made. We've been involved in so many accidents lately, that we know the wrecker driver by name. He used to be a volunteer first responder, so he got almost all of our business. And he's seen the both of us at scenes similar to this one.

We all squish into the front cab of the wrecker, and with Ernie that's a real task. He's literally oozing up against me. I feel like a small ingredient in a sub-sandwich. I could be a pickle slice, or a bit of lettuce. Ernie is all the meat and mustard and mayo. The wrecker is the bun.

Ernie and I have to stop crashing units.

Right now we're tied up at one a piece.

15
OFFICER'S
CLEARINGHOUSE

December 19th
Tuesday, 8:12 am . . .

"*Springfield Dispatch to Metro-EMS . . . we have a possible medical call. Check on well being. Ten-thirteen North Jackson.*"

Ernie and I were shopping for gifts for the *Toys for Tots* program. You know, Ernie and his big heart, he just *had* to volunteer us for it. Us. I had suggested lumps of coal, what with the oil prices what they are, but Ernie gave me a scalding glare as he explained the wonderful things the program does for children. Ernie has a way of making you feel like lumps of cold poop.

If there's a heaven, he's probably got a seat next to Jesus or something. Me, I'm going to have to grease the doorguy just to get past the pearly gates.

We race out, jump in the unit, and head to the scene. We're rolling non-emergency because we don't really have any idea what is going on at this point.

"You don't like kids?" Ernie asks delicately.

I shrug, "Kids are fine. I'm just a grinch."

"Oh," he says, smiling as if that explained everything.

We arrived on the scene, and pull to the side of the street. All that we know is that the guy hasn't spoken to anyone in six or seven days. And his work initiated the 911 call after he had been absent for his fourth consecutive day of work. He's employed at a uniform company and they were worried.

As I bring the unit to a stop we sit there for a moment looking at this old dilapidated house. It's warped old wood with some bricks here and there, white peeling paint, boards hanging dangerously low with exposed rusty nails. This is one of those houses that *Freddy Kruger* would rent. There is plastic covering the windows to keep the cold at bay. And really, this place should have probably been condemned years ago.

The mailbox is stuffed full of sweepstakes envelopes. As it turns out by reading the envelopes, this guy could have already won ten million dollars. So he's got that going for him.

A police Lieutenant, Greg, met us at the front door, and he looked a little pale.

"You look a little flush there, LT," I said with a grin. "You alright?"

He sighed, "This guy's not going to need your help. He needs a mortician, not a paramedic." Then he took a deep breath, his cheeks puffing out as he turned to open the door.

And I mean just the exact second that the door opened we were engulfed by a smell that I still have a hard time describing without feeling sick to my stomach. It's so horrible it turns my insides. I see and touch and smell dead people all the time, but this was different.

Ernie, who never says anything when he's on a scene, he says, "Geez-us Christ! What *is* that?"

Honestly, this smells like the death fart of a large game animal, mixed with an autopsy, multiplied by a hundred. This is one of those levels of hell that my grandmother is always threatening me with.

Disgusting.

We walk into the front hall, and two steps in we could see the body. And it's a mammoth. This enormous fat guy is face down, slowly decomposing on a floor heater. He's naked, except for a thin pair of clearly soiled tighty-whitey underwear. They're so old they're see-through.

Oh, it's just *Pukeville* in here.

See, when somebody dies, all of the muscles in their body eventually relax. But one of the first ones is the sphincter. So add that to the aroma of everything else we're smelling. In this particular case, I think that maybe the underwear were yucky while this pig was alive.

This house is a dreadful mess. Ernie and I look at the body, then turn to the darkness that must have surrounded this guy every waking moment of his life. It's taking some time for our eyes to adjust, and we're actively trying not to vomit all over the place. You can taste this place in the back of your throat.

I wonder if the inside of this guy's place looks anything like the inside of his mind—all dark and decaying and claustrophobic.

Little lines of understanding are starting to form in my mind, connecting cause and effect. The man's face is scratched and chewed-on, and I see cat turds. Somewhere, I figure, angry little felines are running around on a full stomach.

What we have to do now is search for one of two things: *Cause of Death,* or *Mechanism of Injury.* As we're searching, the first thing I see are the stacks upon stacks of sweepstakes entries gathered next to mountains of pornography. And not just dirty pictures, but dirty *everything*.

There are bugs scurrying around, hiding under bigger and more robust items of trash. The window shades are a nicotine-yellow, making sure that no natural light could every find its way into this place. There are unclean dishes and discarded boxes of cereal and crackers. There are empty and half-empty plastic bottles of mustard and mayonnaise. But, curiously, I don't think this guy used them the way I use them.

There are ripped-up pieces of furniture that look like they just gave up and committed suicide, rather than decay due to any feasible wear and tear. I can't think of any scenario where a person could exist in a place like this. There is a spilt box of drywall nails in the middle of the floor near what might be a kitchen. And I can't even begin to ponder what use they served.

This is disgusting beyond comprehension.

"For cause of death," I said, "how about . . . masturbating loser?"

"Should we at least put the pads on him . . . " Ernie asked, "you know, to get a record of his flat line?"

The LT and I both glare incredulously at Ernie. He shrugs and goes back to his search.

We make our way down the cigarette burned hallway, stepping over little land-mines of cat crap, and stop outside the bathroom.

"Whoa!" the Lieutenant says as he backpedals a step or two.

Ernie and I glance at each other, shrug, and then peek inside. There's pornography everywhere. There are two, sticky-looking, rubber anal plugs. There are broken candles, and old fruit, and plastic gloves. There is something that looks like a pearl necklace, but I'm almost certain that it's not meant for anyone's neck.

There is a single brown sandal that looks to have been used for something I can't repeat without an indictment. There is a crumpled towel, cracked and yellow, sitting on top of a knee-high mountain of porno magazines.

On the sink there are several small tubes of medicine. On the left side, near the toilet, there is a large plastic container of hemorrhoid cream and, of course, the lid is nowhere to be found. In the brown-stained bath tub there are several empty, seemingly discarded, bottles of cheap skin cream. I bet one of those purple CSI lights would turn this place so bright your eyes would explode.

Looking at all of this I have no words. This is beyond anything I have ever seen. This is the kind of thing that Hollywood types come up with. It's too real.

"So," Ernie says, breaking the silence that we're all holding on to so preciously, " . . . this is the entertainment center, I guess."

The Lieutenant heads back down the hallway, saying, "You think we ought to move the body? It can't be good leaving him on that floor heater."

"What are those for?" Ernie says pointing naively to the anal plugs.

I laugh to myself, "Nothing, Ernie. Nothing at all."

We head back down the hall, and into the living room. Or I suppose you could call it a dying room. They're both appropriate. I look at this fat, gross, mound of deadness. "I'm not fucking touching that thing," I say sternly. "A coroner should be handling this."

Ernie, who is always trying to do the right thing, bends down and takes a hold of one of the man's legs, right below the knee, and gives it a gentle tug. And like pulling a sock off, the skin sloughs free of the bones.

The whole thing, all at once. A big old flesh sock.

"Holy——" I start.

" . . . *shit!*" the LT finishes.

And Ernie, completely caught off guard by this, falls backwards, crushing all sorts of trash beneath him until he smashes into the wall.

This limp skin sack in his hands, Ernie is looking around uncomprehendingly. "What . . . how did . . . are you kidding?"

We all taste our lunch coming back up, creeping past our throats. This is officially the most disgusting thing . . . *ever.* I'm seconds away from puke, actively fighting my double-cheeseburger back down.

I turn on my heels right then, and march out the front door. I head out to my trusty spot next to the ambulance's exhaust pipe and suck in the beautiful scent of diesel fumes.

Behind me the Lieutenant starts laughing, giving Ernie the business about this maybe being a homicide investigation, and how he's tainting the crime scene.

Ernie, he's pulling a full-on icky dance, high-stepping it to the front door, meeting me by the exhaust pipe. I got some methylated cream to put over my top lip, and gave some to Ernie. Then we marched back inside. The cream gives you a shiny white mustache, but you can't smell anything awful, so it's wonderful.

The LT asks us what we've got on and we answer him. He, naturally, asks for some and we give it to him. He puts a huge line of it right under his nose, sniffing comfortably.

"It's neat that you guys carry this stuff around in the ambulance."

"Oh," I told him. "I didn't get it out of the ambulance, Greg."

"Huh?"

"No, I got it from the bathroom sink."

Ernie and I watch as the Lieutenant's face morphs into something between horror and disbelief. He starts screaming and grunting, pretty much just making yuck noises.

Then he starts to try and wipe what he thinks is dead-guy hemorrhoid cream off his lips with his sleeve. And you know all that's really doing is spreading it out over the rest of his contorted face. This cream is designed to be spread and just soak in.

Now he's in a real panic. He starts barking, "You're lucky you two assholes don't work for me! I'd have fired your asses just for that. God damn it!"

And I think it was at that point that I decided not to tell him the truth—that the cream actually came from my personal pack, and not from the bathroom of horrors.

What a dick. Some people just can't take a joke.

I pick up my radio, glancing at Ernie, "Metro-three is available from the scene. No transport."

And then I slap Ernie on the shoulder, "Let's get out of here before we catch something. I'm starving."

We leave the Lieutenant there. I guess he'll call the coroner and they can arm wrestle over who is going to pull all of the dead guy's skin off trying to move that corpse. They'll never sell that house to anyone else.

No way.

Not ever.

16
WRONG CHEMISTRY

September 17th
Tuesday, 10:34 pm . . .

"Springfield Dispatch to Metro-EMS . . . medical emergency. We have a chemical spill at Grower's Chemicals. Two individuals involved."

Ernie and I just left the McDonalds, with hot fries and sodas and cheeseburgers just waiting for us. I pick up the radio, "Metro-three en route." And off we go.

Grower's Chemical is in an industrial area on the west side of town. They specialize in fertilizer and other agricultural and industrial chemicals. They are constantly receiving train shipments. Those black tanker trucks that you often see on trains are carting around the kinds of nasty chemicals that Grower's uses.

It takes us about six minutes to get to the scene. When we get there the fire department is on scene. They're always available, and because of the sheer number of stations that firefighters have, they are almost always on the scene first. Most firemen are also EMTs with extensive medical training and experience in the field. The firefighters usually secure the scene and begin with the patient care prior to our arrival.

As we pull up, there are a group of firefighters flagging us down, pointing us to the rear of the chemical company.

When we get there, the firefighters have two men under the emergency showers—showers set-up specifically for hazardous spill or emergency chemical exposures. It's freezing cold, and these two pour souls are wearing just jeans. They're standing underneath the cold decontaminating water, shaking almost uncontrollably.

As we're making our way the firefighters tell us the story: The two guys were hooking up a hose in order to start the pump that transfers all the chemical load. For whatever reason, they didn't get a good seal when they were connecting the hose. So, when they turned the pump on it started spraying Anhydrous Ammonia all over the place.

We could still smell it in the air as we approached. These two men had been drenched, and had sustained chemical burns over a large portion of their bodies.

The first thing we're grateful for is that they were under the emergency showers. That flushed away a good deal of the harmful chemicals. What we have to do now is cut them free of their clothes, because their clothes are still contaminated, and are still burning them. At the same time we have to be careful not to let them get hypothermia due to the cold.

We each take one of them. They walk unassisted, but they needed guidance because their eyes are swollen shut by the Anhydrous Ammonia.

I take my patient and sit him on a cot, and Ernie takes his patient inside the unit and sets him on the bench. We both go to work assessing our patients' ABCs. That meant, removing the remainder of their clothes and keeping them warm.

Both of these men are older gentlemen, so we're quick to put them on the cardiac monitor and assess their vitals. We're searching for any signs or symptoms of shock, and calculating the body surface-area burned.

We're worried about hypo-volemic shock—loss of fluid from the circulation that leaks from the damaged area that has lost its protective covering of skin. Burns kill not just by damaging tissue, but also by allowing this leakage of fluids and salts—namely sodium and potassium—which keep the heart pumping.

So we don't want our guys to crash due to the surface area of the burns. We keep a close watch on the monitor, and it's just about as important as any of the other steps of the treatment.

I start to cut away the clothes and they just fall apart like wet toilet paper. The Anhydrous Ammonia had really done a number on them.

Ernie is with his patient, and he's got oxygen helping him breathe. Apparently he's having some problems with the chemicals affecting his lungs.

By early intervention—being hosed down and relieved of the clothes that were continuing to burn them—they most likely prevented permanent damage.

They both sustained burns on over 65% of their body's surface area. Burns greater than 75% are usually lethal. These guys were knockin' on heaven's door, had they been out there any longer.

We start IVs and begin pushing fluids—Lactated Ringer's. We use a burn gel on their skin that continued to neutralize the chemicals. We have both patients in the back of the unit, constantly assessing their conditions while a fireman drives us to the hospital.

I get on the radio to call this in, "Metro-three to Medical Control . . . we're inbound to your facility with two Priority-two traumas. Victims of chemical burn. Upon arrival victims had just been removed from an anhydrous ammonia spill, and had spent fifteen minutes in an emergency shower. Both of the victims have burns to a large amount of of their body surface area."

I glance down at the two men, and quickly to the monitors as I continue, " . . . both of them are in a moderate amount of physical pain. We removed all items of clothing and flushed those areas additionally with water and burn gel. Started large-bore IVs on both for fluid replacement. Both patients are in a comfortable position. We've been following ATLS protocols. Do you have any other questions or orders?"

"Medical Control to Metro-three . . . no questions or orders at this time. We will be expecting your arrival."

And with that we preceded to the hospital where they were handed off to the burn unit staff.

Luckily—I found out a couple years later, while teaching a CPR class at Grower's Chemical—I learned that both men made a full recovery. In fact, it was those two men that were in my CPR class that told me about their recovery.

So that was a pretty good feeling. Plus, they have really good coffee.

17

Terrorist Attack on the Winos

October 22nd
Tuesday, 8:13 am...

The office is quiet as a church. All of the staff are gone for the weekend. We just finished having a nice Sunday breakfast with the fire department. My stomach is stuffed full of eggs and bacon. I'm feeling pretty good right now.

Brian—one of our part-time guys—races in with all sorts of curious items. We have no idea what he's up to, but he's a devious sort of guy, kind of shifty-eyed and always into something. He rushed to the freezer and offloaded whatever it was he had, and told us not to ask any questions, all *Unabomber*-like.

Brian is a young guy, clean cut. He's got blond hair and blue eyes. And he perpetually has that mischievous look about him that lets you know he's always into something untoward. Maybe not illegal, per se, but definitely suspicious.

He promises he'll show us soon enough.

So we go through the tedium of getting all the ambulances washed and re-supplied, just like we do for every shift. As we're finishing up Brian comes out with his brown paper bag and a couple of empty 2-litre bottles.

He's always doing pranks and trickery, so we corner him, "Brian, what's going on?"

He tells us that last night we got a call across the street in the parking garage, and it was none other than Billy Angel, saying something about having maggots in his rectum.

Brian was angry, "That mean old son of a bitch started griping me out for waking *him* up. Him!"

"So," Ernie asked him, "what do you plan to do about that?" And Ernie's not asking as a taunt, but as a genuine query. He'll probably note it in his report or something.

The building across from us is an older area that used to be used for retail. Half of the parking garage has been condemned due to falling chunks of concrete. But bums don't mind the risk. It's like a homeless hotel. Maybe not the safest, but warmer than being in the blasting cold of the downtown nights.

"Well, Ernie . . . I'm going to go and wake them up." Brian gets this evil smirk, "Have you ever seen that show on television called, *Mr. Wizard*? You know, where they teach you about chemical reactions and stuff?"

And we've all seen that show, so we nod like the co-conspirators we've now become.

Brian continues, "Well, we're going to make a couple of dry ice bombs. Then we're going to toss them under the parking garage. Give those guys a little wake-up call."

Note to reader: this is all pre-9/11, so you could still pull crap like this without riding the lightning or ending up in Guantanamo Bay.

We all trade nervous glances. "I hate to be the voice of reason," I say, "but should we really do this? Those people suffer enough, don't they?"

Brian squints at me, "What happened to the Danny Stubbs I met?" He looks around to the others, "Can somebody tell me where Medic-thirteen is?"

"Look," I said, "I'm just saying we need to be careful."

"We're not going to hurt anyone," Brian says calmly. A real smooth talker, that one. He adds, "Remember all the shit Billy Angel has pulled in the last few years."

"*Years!*" Don said incredulously, " . . . in the last few *days*."

We all nod. Brian's good at getting the crowd involved. This is how a riot starts. This is how revolutions begin. How governments are toppled.

"So," I say finally, "what's the plan?"

Dry ice bombs work on this principle: There is a chemical reaction in an enclosed space between aluminum foil and dry ice—solidified carbon dioxide. What occurs is a rapid expansion of gas inside a sealed 2-litre bottle that creates an incredible boom.

A boom fit for Billy Angel!

I guess I need to make an admission here. At this time I am working with Brian today. My old partner

Tim—the Vietnam Vet whack-job—is working with my supervisor Don. Don's stuck with Tim because everybody else refuses to work with him. Kind of like an arranged marriage.

I'm sure that Tim's fellow soldiers in Vietnam probably felt the same way we all do about him. Heck, maybe that's how he burned his head.

Well, right now Tim is asleep in one of the staff bedrooms, counting Vietcong, or land mines, or whatever it is he dreams about. But that never occurs to me.

We lay out all of the bomb-making parts, just like good little *Jihadiis*, and assemble our improvised devices. This feels *so* wrong that I know it *has* to be right.

Once the bombs are built we run them across the street and strategically place them inside the parking garage. We don't throw them too far in because they might end up hurting somebody. And then we'd get stuck having to take care of them.

Our explosives set, we sprint back across the street and run back to the safety of the garage, using the ambulances for cover. We're expecting big things. At any moment a large order detonation should thunder in all directions.

Windows will break.

Bums will run in every direction.

It will be wonderful!

And we wait. And we continue waiting. Brian assures us that it will happen, just give it some time. Two minuets go by. Then three. Four. Five.

"Brian are you sure that—"

He holds up a warning finger, "Just be patient."

Six minutes. Still nothing.

Seven minutes.

And now we're all of the mindset that nothing is going to happen. This is a huge letdown. This must be how terrorists feel when their bombs don't go off. What a downer.

Maybe it's because of how the buildings are aligned. Or perhaps it's the location, or the concrete, or just, I don't know what. But when those puppies finally *do* explode, it's like the end of the world.

Ka-booom!

Ka-boooooom!

They went off one after the next, as if we'd had Mr. Wizard make them himself. Every one of us jumped.

The bums got up right away, and they looked like a bunch of freaked out zombies. Like in Michael Jackson's *"Thriller"* video. And they're just bumping into each other, going in every direction with no real plan. It's beautiful, delicious chaos.

And it was scripted by us, those loving paramedics who live right across the street. Don, as animated as I've ever seen him, said, "Shooooooo," gritting his teeth, kind of half fretting, half smiling at the same time.

We start to hear a bunch of shuffling and crashing going on in one of the back rooms. And it's coming from where the staff bedrooms are located. Hmmm?

"Who's back there?" Ernie asks as we run toward the crew quarters.

We're thinking we might have injured somebody it was so loud. I mean, anything could have happened. So, we're *shitting-in-our-pants-scared* right now. We don't say it, but it's going through all of our minds, we might have killed somebody.

Don and I look at each other, and we both say, "Tim."

We open the door to the bedroom where the racket is coming from. And we see this large ass and legs sticking out from under the bed. This is the most depressingly funny thing I've ever seen.

Tim is stuck, wedged under the bed, trying to climb farther under it for cover. He's a total freaking lunatic. And the first thing somebody says is,

"Look what you did *now*, Brian."

We all cross our arms and look at him like he's *David Koresh* or *Jim Jones*, or *Oprah*. One of those people who spin your mind all around and makes you follow their instructions like a mindless zombie. Grab that knife. Drink that juice.

I'm so glad that none of this was my idea. Because I really feel like crap. What we should be doing right now is helping Tim. Telling him the war hasn't started again, and that he's alright. We should be getting him out from under that tiny bed, and calming his racing nerves. Something to comfort the guy.

But instead what we do is go out by the wash bays and laugh uncontrollably until we we're crying. Most of us were on the floor, clutching our chests because we were having a hard time breathing. It was that funny. As scared as Tim was, it was that level of hilarity. We'll probably all rot in hell for that one day. That one moment.

And it will have been worth it.

Then we all get silenced as the radio comes alive, *"Springfield Dispatch to Metro-EMS . . . got a report of a disturbance in the area of your station."*

And now we're all clenching our teeth.

Don, being the supervisor, and only sensible adult, clears his throat and replies, "This is Metro-EMS . . . Negative, uh, we haven't seen anything. Just, uh, maybe a car backfire."

There were complaints from the homeless guys. But they fell on deaf ears. The cops asked us a few questions that we successfully dodged. We were basically unscathed.

But Gary—the director—did eventually come down on us. We got reprimanded about not being sensitive to other employee's emotional needs. Particularly Tim's. He wasn't so much mad about the bums or the bombs. Just the fact that we'd caused Tim to go nuthouse crazy.

"Tough love, boss," I said at the meeting. "It's just our way of telling him we care."

18

BODIES
EVERYWHERE

November 23rd
Saturday, 12:38 pm . . .

"Springfield Dispatch to Metro-EMS . . . injury accident, Seventy-one Highway, exit thirty-two. We have multiple nine-one-one calls. Springfield Fire is en route, as well as Rural Fire."

Ernie and I were just fueling up at the "pumps" when we heard the call. I keyed-up and responded, "Medic-twenty-three, this is Medic-thirteen . . . we can respond to that call. We're at the pumps."

I then hear my supervisor call to dispatch, *"Metro-EMS to Springfield Dispatch . . . Metro-four and Metro-seven en route. Please put LifeFlight on standby."*

Today Ernie and I are in Metro-four. It's a brand new slope-side, Powerstroke Turbo-diesel. And this puppy is fast! Crazy fast. *Shoot your wife and lead the cops on a high-speed chase to Mexico fast!*

Once we get on it, we can feel the power of the engine pressing us back against our seats. Stuff was flying by so fast that I thought we were jumping to hyperspace.

"Can't this thing go any faster?" Ernie says facetiously.

I'd give him a glance if I didn't think we'd crash at these speeds. "Ernie," I tell him, " . . . if we go any faster we'll travel into the future."

Nine minutes later we're arriving onto the scene, and the whole way there we had been hearing the radio chatter and all the various people giving their takes on the madness. And this is what we've distilled thus far: A drunk driver had a collision with an old pick-up, maybe a Chevy. The pick-up had one of those camper shells over the bed. And there's bits scattered all over the place. Like a bomb went off.

Some guy even got on the radio, saying, "We've got patients everywhere!" And he didn't sound like he was acting. You can tell when you listen to people on the radio long enough if they're shocked, or just playing it up. What we were hearing was that this was devastating.

Our supervisor puts another ambulance en route due to the sheer number of patients. LifeFlight was given the order to launch. And it was all a chaotic mess.

Immediately upon our arrival we begin to triage the patients, making determinations about who needs the most urgent care and in what order. The first thing I notice about the scene was that it looks like a plane crash. There is debris everywhere. Bits of plastic and chunks of metal, some shredded blankets, children's toys, broken glass, papers, and just about everything you can imagine.

This is like looking at the inside of somebody's house, discarded on a triangular stretch of banked grass between a highway entrance and an access road.

The wreckage is scattered over an area of more than a hundred meters in every direction.

A volunteer firefighter briefly explains, "There was a family of five coming into town to do some early Christmas shopping. This drunk driver, he basically crossed the median and struck the family's vehicle head-on, in the driver's side quarter. The father was probably dead on impact. The wife is smashed to pieces, but she's alive. She's in the vehicle, still. Drunk driver is still in his vehicle."

And then he swallowed, taking a breath, " . . . the, uh, children, they . . . all three of them were ejected from the shell like small missiles."

By the time he finishes giving us the rundown, the second ambulance is arriving. I tell him to set-up the LZ for the LifeFlight helicopter.

My assessment is this: Because of the mechanism of injury—the death of the father—we have five Priority-1 patients. Each one gets their own medic and firemen as they arrive. There is, thankfully, an overwhelming amount of help here.

A fireman yells, "This one's got a pulse!" So I run over to this small girl.

Ernie grabs a kid about 15 feet away from me. But we had to hunt through the grass and broken debris to find them. My patient was a little girl, maybe 9 years old. I glance back, noticing that we were at least 35 yards away from the accident. There was a toolbox next to her, and I think she might have gotten hit by it during the crash.

I have my Airway bag already. The Airway bag has the following instruments and tools: Oxygen, oral airways (simple airway adjuncts that allow quick airway access, used prior to endotracheal intubation), endotracheal tubes, a laryngoscope (lifts the tongue and jaw out of the way so the medic can visualize the entrance of the trachea), the BVM with oxygen reservoir, bite blocks, stylettes (pieces of wire used to help shape the endotracheal tube for better insertion), and a sphygmomanometer (blood-pressure cuff).

This little girl that I'm looking at has shoulder-length blond hair, with a blue *Pokemon* sweater, and blue jeans. When I assessed her I had to check her eyes. With a head injury the patient will most often get one dilated eye, and one constricted pupil. I noticed that her eyes were the most intense color of green as I pull her eyelids back. Sure enough, one of her eyes is extremely dilated.

Brilliant, but vacant.

Behind me Ernie is calling for all of his equipment. Firefighters are running to the unit to fetch his gear. Other firemen are holding in-line stabilization on all of the patients.

I inserted an oral airway on the little girl and started breathing. This is just a temporary fix until I can get to the unit and intubate her. She had a shattered jaw and I assume that's where something heavy made contact with her. We get her packaged-up—C-collar, towel rolls, backboard. As we're doing this we notice that the LifeFlight helicopter is landing in the middle of the highway. It looks like they're loading up the mother and one of the children.

Ernie and I get our patients ready about the same time. We load both children onto gurneys and head for the unit, firemen assisting us every step of the way. Once we arrive at the units, we get the children in the back as quickly as possible. There is a fireman behind the wheel, just waiting for an order.

We see one of the other ambulances take off with the drunk driver. Our second ambulance was helping the LifeFlight helicopter get loaded-up and briefed.

Everything is happening all at once. From above, this probably looks like a bunch of ants racing around, systematically dealing with some major catastrophe. No wasted motion. No time for pondering and indecision. No pause, not even for a second.

This is order out of chaos.

Evolution.

The total scene time was probably less than 12 minutes. You see, from the instant of any accident the clock starts ticking. You have the Golden Hour to save your patient. Time starts running out from the beginning of that Golden Hour. That's what they teach you, anyway.

The reality is that we have a Golden *15 minutes*.

Ernie and I go to work inside the back of the unit, assisted by one of the firemen. Ernie has fastened his patient down on the bench. I've got the little girl on the cot. The fireman is helping us in any way he can, carefully staying out of the way, but close enough to assist when we request.

We both intubate our patients. On the little girl I have to do a very difficult procedure, a nasal intubation —from the nose to the trachea. I get lucky, though, and the tube goes right in.

Ernie's patient vomited, so he had to unstrap him from the bench and turn him—still taped to his backboard—onto his side and clear the airway again. I handed him the suction so he could clear out the airway.

The suction has a really long tube that attaches near me, and I notice that the tube is filled with blood. Ernie's patient isn't doing so well. I say *patient* instead of *dying child*. It's easier to rationalize it like that.

The fireman in the back set up all the IV bags with drip sets for us. I check the monitor to make sure that the little girl had a good rhythm, and a good *bounding* —strong—pulse. I then hand off the BVM to the fireman so that I can start an IV on her. Once the IV was in place I start pushing fluids.

Ernie was setting up his IV at the same time. We're like synchronized swimmers.

I make sure that Ernie has everything going on his patient, then I look up to make sure the fireman is driving us in the right direction. We took care of all the life threats. I could hear LifeFlight and Metro-seven calling in their radio reports.

I then reassessed our patients, gathering as much information as possible. Ernie gives me a short summary of his patient's status so I can thoroughly inform the hospital of what to expect. It sounds like, listening to the other radio reports, that everybody's got their hands full.

When I finally call in my radio report, I first want to know if the hospital is prepared to accept three more Priority-1 trauma patients. If they take three patients then they will need three emergency room trauma teams. That's a lot of people.

I also need to make sure that the hospital's MRI machine is functioning because we are dealing with head injuries. All of these things are cascading through my mind right now.

Immediately when I start my radio report they divert us to another hospital. It was roughly the same distance away. Same ETA. It wouldn't make much of a difference in time on the road, but it would be much better for the patients.

We pretty much do everything we can. We continue to check the ABC's over and over. You always have to reassess.

Airway.

Check.

Breathing.

Check.

Circulation.

Check.

Airway . . . and you keep on doing it. This continuous cycle never stops. You can't miss it even one time. Two minutes without checking is one minute and fifty-nine seconds too long.

The little girl I'm working on isn't getting any worse. But then, she isn't improving either. With head injuries, a strange thing can happen. The patient's heart rate can start to lower while their blood pressure shoots up. This is one of the signs of increased inner-cranial pressure. And the pressure may be a result of inner-cranial bleeding. It's crowded in the head, up there. There's not a lot of room for *extra* fluids floating around.

Within minutes we drop the little girl and boy off at the hospital, delivering them into the arms of the emergency room trauma team. Your typical trauma team consists of a bunch of people—surgeons, nurses, radiology, everybody. And once the patients are turned over, that's it for us. We make our reports and keep out of the way.

Ernie and I walk back out to the unit and start cleaning. I call the supervisor on the radio, "Metro-four to Metro-one . . . Metro-four is going to be out-of-service. En route to station to replenish supplies and clean-up."

"Copy that, Metro-four. Return to station."

We don't stand around wondering about our patients. They aren't ours anymore. We had to get back, get the unit ready, and head back out to answer more calls. We don't get much down time.

Thing is, people are always getting shot, or in wrecks, or falling off of stuff they shouldn't be on. And they don't wait for us to get *ready* when they do it.

Later, I found out that the mother made it. But the other child in the LifeFlight helicopter didn't. The child that Ernie had been working on pulled through. But my patient, the cute little girl with the dazzling green eyes, she crashed in the emergency room.

The only positive thing that came of it was that her organs were viable for donors. While it's no consolation for the mother who lost two children and her husband in a matter of an instant, it's at least nice to know that several other children might be saved with those organs.

I don't know if that's a silver lining or not. Lemons out of lemonade?

It is what it is.

19
GO-CART JUMP START

May 10th
Saturday, 2:53 pm . . .

"Springfield Dispatch to Metro-EMS . . . we have a call of an unresponsive person at Sixty-six Go-cart Speedway."

My supervisor, Don, is working with me today. And we just happen to be at the Sprint-car Speedway, right next door, standing-by in case there are any medical emergencies. We thought it would be an easy extra shift to work. Race cars, girls, nachos, that kind of thing.

For the last two hours we had been sitting with a bunch of fire and safety officials, watching the sprint cars get sideways and kick up dust on the big, hard-packed, dirt oval track. At time-and-a-half overtime pay, this isn't a bad way to spend a Saturday.

Don keys-up, "Metro-eight to Springfield Dispatch . . . Metro-eight copies direct. We're going to respond from the regular speedway."

It actually takes us four or five minutes to disentangle ourselves from the regular speedway. Since we were being paid to be there, we have to call a replacement unit to cover our position while we go next door.

We hop in the unit, and race a half mile down the road to the *Go-cart Speedway*, and we see some of the crowd, flagging us down. We get out, grab all of our gear, throwing it on the gurney. We know we're going to need it if the guy's coding.

We're not at one of those grandma-grandpa kinds of go-cart tracks with candy and popcorn. No, these are privately-owned go-cart racing teams. These suckers can fly over a 100 miles per hour. This is serious stuff.

"He's right over here," some guy says. "We think he's dead!"

They say that he started talking funny, saying some "*weird shit,*" and then he went out. And that was that.

We pass all of the pit crews, several fences, and then we see our patient. There is a guy laying down, in full racing attire—leather suit, helmet, gloves, and boots.

So we drop all of our stuff. Don went to his head and removed his helmet. He had on an open-faced, half-skull helmet. He's checking his airway.

I'm pulling the guy's suit down so that I can apply the fast-patches. Some firemen that had arrived about the same time as us are actually cutting his suit. I use scissors to cut his t-shirt so that I can get the fast-patches on.

Once I get him up on the monitor I notice that he's in V-fib (Ventricular fibrillation). On the monitor that looks like a bunch of squiggly lines because the heart is quivering instead of correctly firing.

"Don, he's in V-fib," I say. "We've got to shock him right away!"

Don has just gotten an oral airway in, but he backs off, dropping the BVM so that I can administer the shock. You can hear an audible whine as it charges and then I give the shock.

The man's body lifts, it drops, and we're back at it.

Don intubates the man and continues to breathe for him while I reassess the monitor. He's still in V-fib at this point. And everybody has stopped whatever they were doing, and now we're the only show. The race, that's this guy fighting for his life. A race against time.

I increase the joules to 300 and we shock the patient again. What's actually happening when we shock the heart is that we're stopping all heart function, and resetting it, again. So, you're not starting the heart, your stopping it so that it can start itself.

We clear our hands and I administer the shock. The man lifts awkwardly off the ground, and then drops back down. And lo and behold, it's worked.

I say, "We have normal sinus rhythm, Don."

And the crazy thing is, even though the heart's electrical activity is back to normal, there is *still* no pulse. This can happen. It's known as PEA—*Pulseless Electrical Activity*.

So, we're not out of the woods.

I go to start an IV while Don finishes tying down the endotracheal tube. He lets a fireman continue the breathing while he reaches over and cracks open the drug box. Each drug box has a numbered seal on it for accountability's sake.

Don draws up some epinephrine and he checks me to see if I've started the IV.

"No, we've got no veins," I say. The problem I'm having is that when there's no pulse, and no good pressure, the veins go flat. What it means is that I might have to try the femoral or jugular veins. But that takes time. Valuable time that we may not have.

Don administers the epinephrine via the endotracheal tube. It's a small dosage, at a high concentration, and is actually shot directly into the tube. It's the fastest route other then venous to administer a drug. The patient will actually aspirate the epinephrine.

At this point I've found my landmark—the proper site for chest compressions—and crack his sternum as I began the chest compressions. That is an awful sound to the uninitiated.

The crowd goes *ooooh!* as they hear the crunch.

I'm continuing to do chest compressions. The fireman is handling the BVM. We're continuing CPR to allow the epinephrine to circulate through the system. This is our emergency medical symphony.

While this is happening, Don is calling the hospital to ask Medical Control if they have any instructions. We tell them we're on the scene. He informs them of the patient's condition and our treatment up to this point.

Medical Control asks us to administer Atropine Sulfate as is indicated per ACLS. They want us to continue all ACLS protocols until further indicated.

The Atropine Sulfate is supposed to assist the epinephrine in stimulating the heart muscle into reanimating. So that's what we do.

I finally got an IV in the femoral vein, and that's where we introduced the Atropine Sulfate.

The fireman yells, "He's got a pulse!"

And the crowd starts to cheer and celebrate. And really it scared the piss out of me because I had forgotten that we were surrounded by a bunch of onlookers. When you start working on a patient, you forget about everything else around you.

This was like some cheesy made-for-TV moment. People are patting each other on the shoulders. Congratulatory slaps on the back. High-fives. Democrats and Republicans hugging each other. Dogs and cats living together.

While this is erupting around us we begin to package-up the patient. This guy still needs the hospital and all of their wonder and magic to stabilize him.

Bear in mind that this guy is still lights-out. When we have a clinical save such as this, the patient rarely gains consciousness like they do on TV. This is the real world. And the reality is that we've only gotten his heart working again. He still may not ever gain consciousness. He might end up a vegetable, or crash five minutes from now.

But try explaining *that* to a smiling, joyous crowd of 3,000 people, some of them all teary-eyed and crying. Good luck.

We just let them think the best. Give them their happy ending. A story they can tell over dinner the next couple nights.

Our job is only just beginning. We have to get this patient to the hospital. There, doctors can do extensive testing to determine the underlying cause of what happened, and take this guy off of our hands so that we could get back to the races.

We get him packaged-up, up on a gurney, and out to the unit quickly. Before long we are racing down the highway, me at the wheel, making the radio report; Ernie in the back with the still unconscious patient. Within six minutes we've delivered him to the emergency room staff, and are back in the unit, heading for the track.

I've got money on the number 68 sprint car, and his main race hasn't started yet. Patients are like stinger missiles: Fire and forget. Once they're out of your hands, it's like it never happened.

The demons and ghosts . . . they wait until the darker hours to start haunting us. Maybe in the middle of the night when I get up for a glass of water, I'll see one of them out of the corner of my eyes. They don't say much. They just walk on by, their eyes completely black from the 8-ball hemorrhages. Maybe they're missing an arm, or filled with stab wounds.

A couple *Xanax* later . . . they're gone.

20
WISE GUY

November 4ᵗʰ
Tuesday, 1:00 pm ...

'On Call ... *report to station for delta transfer!*'

A delta transfer is a long distance, non-emergency, patient transfer. This is a very common, ordinary procedure, and we do about three of these a day. They can be transfers of anywhere between 30 and 300 miles of travel. We do this with patients who might be in a medical facility in another town, that now need to return to a closer facility. We might transfer nursing home patients, or certain patients who are going to get a very specialized medical procedure.

I slide on my boots, jump in my Ford Ranger, and within minutes I'm skidding to a stop in the station parking lot. When I get there I'm met by Rob—a senior crew chief—who has been waiting for me. Let me tell you about Rob. He might just be the ugliest man on the face of the earth.

He's got piercing blue eyes that draw you to his ugliness. He's average-sized, balding, with a hefty gut. He has back problems, like most paramedics. He's got this annoying way he talks, somewhere between a whistle and a whine. And he's even uglier than Tim, which I would have never thought possible. His years of experience have weighed down his jowls, sagging his flanks like a bulldog.

But unlike Tim, he has an air of wisdom about him. He's almost sagely. He is highly respected among the other paramedics because he's seen and done a lot. And there is no substitute for experience. So when he talks, a smart man will listen.

Rob knows about the animosity between Tim and I. I kind of think that Tim and Rob are friends and he wants to mediate some kind of truce, or understanding, between us. We do spend a third of our lives together, and it would be best if we figured out some way to coexist.

We clock-in, grab the drug box keys, get assigned our unit by the supervisor working, and then we head out to the ambulance. The whole time Rob is talking to me in this kind of friendly fatherly way.

We're en route to La Grange, 75 miles to the south, to pick-up a nursing home patient for dialysis —the process of removing blood from a patient whose kidney functioning is faulty, purifying that blood, and returning it to the patient's bloodstream.

This should be a relaxing drive both ways, with little or no stress involved. In this case, Rob was driving, taking his time as he began to explain to me lessons that he'd learned over the many years he's been working.

"I've been a crew chief for many years, Danny," he starts.

And this is one of those conversations where I should basically just keep my mouth shut and try to learn from his insights.

" . . . I've been to a lot of calls, and seen a lot of, well," and he shook his head back and forth as he sighed through his nose, "just awful things. You know, when a man sees enough accident scenes, he's really seen the face of humanity. But at its worst, you see. At our most frail and delicate moments. When we're all broken and bent and bleeding, that's when we see the sadness and preciousness of life. That's when we're most vulnerable."

And I glance at my watch. I'm not trying to be rude. I don't really even mean to. I just do it, kind of unconsciously. I see him glancing at me, noticing.

"Really, Danny. We get to see a part of ourselves in each of our patients. And that means that we learn about ourselves from each and every call."

I nod. Nodding, my ex-girlfriend told me, is good because it makes people think you're paying attention. But nodding alone isn't enough. Of course, she tells me all of this as she's explaining why she doesn't want to see me anymore. And to be honest, I forgot most of what she was saying. She was rattling on about paying her more attention or something. You know how girl-friends can be.

Rob gets us onto the highway for the longest, most boring part of the drive, and he continues, "And you know, we learn as much from one another as we do from the patients. We become greater because of our differences. That's the way this country got started. It's a melting pot of interesting and uniquely different people. And we all become better because of those contrasting traits."

I nod again. I'm thinking of a song I like, right now. And when I'm occasionally nodding to the beat in my head, I'm scoring *listening points* with Rob. My ex said the nod was very important positive reinforcement for the speaker.

" . . . I've seen a lot of medics come and go," he says, passing a small 4-door station wagon. "Some of them were good paramedics. Some of them were downright terrible. I mean the worst of the worst. You wouldn't want them to hand you an ace bandage."

I really nod this time because I figure he's talking about Tim.

" . . . some of them left being paramedics and went on to med school, eventually becoming doctors. Some of my old partners are now working with medical supply companies, making the big bucks."

Now, just to change it up, I shake my head slowly. My girlfriend never taught me this, I actually read it in a magazine. You shake your head as if you just can't believe it. It's good for making the speaker think you're *really* into what he's talking about.

"But then," he continues, " . . . it can go the other way, too. Some people leave this job worse off then when they signed-on. They see things that get stuck in their head. They're stubborn. They're disrespectful of those around them. With every success story there is a sad tale of somebody who fell apart. I had an ex-partner who went to prison."

And I don't say it, but I'm thinking *drugs*. This job is so stressful that it sends people to recreational drug use. And from there, well, things have a way of spiralling out of control.

For a second I'm wondering if he's going to give me the *get help for your habit* speech. You know, the one where he is all understanding and compassionate about why I turned to the alcohol, the weed, the cocaine, and the prescription medicines. I've actually been preparing myself for a speech like that for months, now.

"I guess what I'm trying to say is, we have to be less judgemental about our partners."

Whew! Dodged a bullet there.

" . . . we have to understand that all of those differences between us, that might rub us the wrong way, those are the things we should be patient with. We all have to live together, you know."

"This is about Tim, isn't it?" I ask. But I'm not really asking.

"Yes and no. It is about you and Tim, only because I know there's a lot of friction there. But it is also referring to all of us, and the people we work with now, and in the future. You won't always be working here, or maybe you will. Who knows? But we all have to be in an environment that we can function to the best of our abilities. At the end of the day, it is about saving human lives."

I have to resist the temptation to bash Tim right now. He's the worst medic in history, but I'm sure

Rob knows that. "I always put the job first," I say to him as I turn and stare out the window.

And a slight smile passes across Rob's otherwise serious face, "I heard about the dry-ice bombs."

Oh.

"That man went stark crazy trying to hide under that bed."

"It was an unfortunate side effect of our antics," I say, my eyes looking down to simulate regret. "And I'm not proud of it."

And the Oscar for best performance in an ambulance goes to . . .

"You know Tim has had a difficult time readjusting since the war," Rob says as if it happened yesterday. As if he just got back from Iraq.

"The *war* was Vietnam. He was in-country *thirty* years ago," I pointed out. "He's had plenty of time to cope. He's messed-up, Rob. Bigtime. And I don't think he'll ever get over it. This isn't the right job for a guy like that."

I'm saying everything I can without calling him a horribly unsafe medic and attacking his disturbing tendencies to inappropriately touch patients.

Rob nods, and I'm wondering which kind of nod it is. We drive on in silence for the next 40 or 50 minutes and we see a *Dairy Queen* located conveniently next to the nursing home.

"Hungry?" Rob asks as he slows us for the exit.

"Starving," I say. "I could eat a horse cut in half." And that's not a figure of speech because Ernie and I have actually done that.

We order some burgers and grab a table. We need full stomachs for the drive back. Soon enough we are chewing on hot french fries, sipping Coke, and biting into delicious cheeseburgers.

There's some sappy elevator music in the background and I can feel his wisdom coming.

Rob swallows a bit and leans back, "You have to be prepared in this business. That's the most important thing, I think. You must be ready for the task at hand. The demon is in the details, as they say."

"Demons. Yes," I say, shoveling fries into my mouth like they might never serve them after today. We finish our meals and get back to the unit.

Five minutes later we're pulling up to the nursing home. As we get out and head around to the back of the unit he tells me, "Take it easy on Tim, eh. Us old guys, we might have a couple of wires loose, but we're always ready for the call. *Always* prepared!"

And then he opens the back doors and we realize that there's no cot. Therefore, there is no way to transport our patient. And the reason there is no cart is because Rob, I guess, forgot to load it. A cot, that's like the most important part of the transport equation.

"Rob . . . " I say, turning slowly to him, "where's the cot?"

And do you know what *Mr. Always Prepared* had to say? He said, "Hmmm?"

Hmmm? Are you fucking kidding me? But out loud I said, "Well, this complicates things, doesn't it."

Luckily, or unluckily, the woman we came to transport could walk on her own, so we were able to load her up into the jump seat. I elected to stay in the back with her, Rob behind the wheel. This lady's elevator doesn't stop at every floor. So I've got a crazy lady in the back beside me, and a crazy man behind the wheel.

I'd say this is about par for the course.

21
STATION-ARY

December 8th
Monday, 1:02 am . . .

The turf battle between Metro-EMS and Willard County Ambulance Service is at full speed. This is our cold war, and there's no detente.

The state courts eventually got involved with the dispute and they heard the arguments and complaints from both sides. In their infinite wisdom they delivered a landmark ruling. And their determination was that we should both share the same area of the city for emergency response.

For us, this was bigger than *Roe v. Wade*. More outrageous than the *O.J. Simpson* verdict—the not-guilty of murder verdict, not the one in Vegas where he got life for stealing some football cards. For us, this thing was a huge loss. Epic.

You see, ambulance turf battles are as old as ambulances themselves. As old as the sun.

This goes back to that old television show *Emergency*. If you don't remember, it was a daytime television drama based on the adventures of two fire department paramedics. That show changed everything because shortly thereafter, every town in America wanted a paramedic service like that.

Quite suddenly, paramedics and ambulance services popped up everywhere. This is still a non-traditional, very young profession. And with this burgeoning new field came competition. Ambulance services are a lot more like taxis or wrecker services. Most of them are privately-owned, and that creates all kinds of scenarios where hijinks and shenanigans run amuck.

The turf battles naturally evolved from this kind of direct competition. Personal vendettas were just the natural result of the friction. I mean, we're only human.

This court decision gave Willard County Ambulance Service permission to respond to calls in *our* area. This part of the city was now a shared territory. A green zone. Our service's response was to set-up a satellite station in this part of the city—the west side.

The idea was that we would now be able to more quickly respond to calls, and we would beat Willard County to the scene every time. We were cheating within the rules.

This satellite station only required one crew to man it, and tonight that crew is Ernie and me. It doesn't take much to keep it running. The station is basically a simple building with a covered garage for the ambulance to keep the medication and equipment warm. There is a small day room with a kitchenette built into it. Past that is the crew sleeping quarters— two rooms—and then the exit out the front door.

In the two bedrooms there are televisions, beds, a small dresser, a bathroom with shower and sink and toilet, and a small closet for our clothes. It's fairly self-sufficient, and the place is conveniently located less than a minute's walk from a local hospital.

Ernie and I had just finished a patient transfer and we had already cleaned-up the unit. Now we were settling down. We figured we were pretty much done for the night. I'm laying on my bed watching TV while Ernie is in his room. He's most likely eating and reading the bible. He has one of those sleep apnea machines that forces air into his lungs so that he can get a decent night's sleep. Without it he's a gurgling, choking, hacking monster. You listen to him try to sleep without it and you'll lose your lunch.

After about 20 minutes of flipping through the infomercials I hear a subtle knock at my door. I figure Ernie's got some problem, or maybe somebody walked in needing assistance. It happens every now and again, some busted-up prostitute sees our sign and figures we're a clinic.

I sit up, checking my radio to make sure the battery is still good and that I didn't miss a call. But no, it's fine. I get up and walk to the door, opening it as I yawn. And what I see is the exact opposite of my fat, good-hearted, sleep-challenged partner.

I'm staring at a pair of sensuous blue eyes with blond shoulder-length hair. I'm seeing a pair of big brown eyes, luscious lips, and brown hair pulled back into a ponytail. They're both wearing their scrubs—

which, as I recall, are incredibly easy to take off. And they're both looking at me with *that* look.

It's Heather and Megan. And it's like a gift from the heavens.

My mind is flashing back to our last encounter in the jacuzzi. The warm water, their naked bodies, all sorts of wonderful, slippery things. And then I swallow.

Right as I open my mouth to speak Heather pushes me slowly backwards while Megan closes and locks the door behind her. Then they both push me down onto the tiny bed. Megan goes to work on my pants while Heather pulls off my boots. And I kind of don't really know what's going on because all of the blood in my body has flowed away from my head.

Can't . . . form . . . rational . . . thought.

These aggressive little vixens strip me naked and then they pull off their green scrubs in an instant. And they begin to go down on me, one at a time, taking me into their mouth. They alternate, one of them swallowing me up and riding up and down until I'm at the point of explosion, and then suddenly they switch; like they have some special sense about what my limits are.

After they torture me with this wonderful ecstasy for what seems like an eternity, they take it to the next level. And I realize a funny thing: Whenever I'm doing other stuff, I'm thinking about sex. But once I'm actually having sex, or fooling around with two beautiful naked nurses, I have to concentrate on anything *but* sex in order to survive.

Because I don't want to screw this up. I have a reputation to uphold.

See, in a situation like this, if you actually stop and consider how good it feels, and what is going on between the three of you—all naked and writhing and touching and licking and tasting—then you can't last more than a minute. If you think about the pleasure you're experiencing, it's legs shaking, then *goosh-spurt-spurt*, and you're done. Then it's all about making excuses. And I *don't* want to be *that* guy.

So I'm thinking about anything other than this incredible threesome I'm engaged in like a porn star. I'm thinking of race cars, and tool sets, and lawn mowers. And we all become the 6-legged monster for the next few hours. We do things to each other that *Ron Jeremy* and *Jenna Jameson* would be proud of.

And when we all finally climax, it's galactic!

After it's all over, we're cozied up together in the small bed, just catching our breath. And I'm thinking, *Shit, I can't tell anyone about this because we'll all get fired.* I mean, as a guy, this is like one of the top accomplishments a man can ever experience.

Dare I say, an *accolade*.

But we're all so completely fired if I mention so much as a whisper of this to anyone. This is *really* not what you're supposed to be doing when you are one half of the only paramedic team in the station. But in the context of the turf war, I am now the supreme ruler of the earth. Well, of Springfield anyway.

And the reason is clear when I ask Megan about her fiancé.

"Oh," she whispers while her fingers play on my chest, "he's fine. You know, they're really busy, lately. I don't see him that much."

Interestingly enough, Megan's fiancé happens to be a supervisor at Willard County Ambulance Service. I might as well be sleeping with *Helen of Troy*. I could be *Paris*. So, most likely, I've got a nice spot in the pits of eternal damnation waiting for me. *Dante* wrote about my kind.

But, you know, what's a guy to do in a situation like that?

This threesome, it wasn't just about me . . . it was for all of us. It was for every guy out there that doesn't get to roll around with two hot nurses. For every paramedic who's overworked and underpaid. This was for each and every man who has not experienced the forbidden fruit.

So you see, this wasn't *my* threesome. It was greater than that. This was the *people's* threesome.

We laid in that bed for at least another hour, basking in the post-coital bliss and glow. It's really hard not to smile right now as I'm cuddled by these two sensuous bodies. And the icing on the cake is that this day, December 8th, it's my birthday. How nice a gift is that?

"Happy Birthday," Megan whispers in my ear.

22
SMELL SHOCK

March 16th
Monday, 10:12 am . . .

"Springfield Dispatch to Metro-EMS . . . we have a medical emergency on the Safeway construction site on Airport Parkway. We have two men down, possible electrocution."

We're all sitting in the day room when the call comes. Ernie jumps up, "Come on, Danny, let's go! We haven't had a good trauma in two weeks." So that's us getting volunteered. I was the crew chief, but Ernie was the more experienced medic, so it kind of evens out that neither of us is really the boss.

And looking at his sincere, chubby face, who would I be to turn him down at a time like this? So I sigh, get up, and jog in the wake of Ernie, drafting to the ambulance. If I chunked my clipboard at him, I bet it would fall into an orbit around his midsection.

Once on board I radio that we were on our way. As we pull outside it's rainy and miserable. A horrible day for construction, but a good day for electrocution. The environment is perfect.

We head over to the construction site, and we're there in less than eight minutes. Fire and rescue are already on the scene when we arrive.

The workers are about halfway through with the construction of a new supermarket; bits of exposed metal, sheetrock, and brick in every direction.

We're led into the side of the building, walking around scaffolding and loose equipment. Both firetrucks are parked near one section of scaffolding that is located near a telephone pole that is currently arcing, shooting sparks and bright flashes everywhere. I notice that everyone is standing in mud as the firemen try to get the power shut off. Electrical conductivity is a fairly simple principle to understand.

Nobody but me seems to mind that we're all sitting in a perfect electrical trap. As I get closer I see that the fire captain has gotten the electricity shut down, using fiberglass pike poles to keep the lines under control.

When it's safe he gives us the wave, "I got it fellas, come on in."

On a three-story section of scaffolding we have two patients, one on the top level, one on the second level. And they're both down. It smells like burnt dog hair. Only, I don't see any dogs, and last I checked they didn't have dogs working on construction sites, something about union rules.

I'm talking to the fire captain who arrived on the scene first. Quickly, he explains, "These guys were working on the scaffolding and they were told by the power company that these lines were dead. One guy found out, real quick, that they weren't dead. And then his *buddy* must have tried to pull him free, and he got it pretty bad. They're both unresponsive, and they're both still on the scaffolding."

Yeesh!

On the top level there is an employee and a firefighter kneeling over one of the patients. On the second level there are three firemen kneeling down. There are people everywhere, but they're all jammed up into the smallest possible space.

I order the firemen near us to get the backboards and the gurney from the ambulance, and I climb up to the very top level. On the way up I see one guy with a fireman working on him and I know that's where Ernie is going. I yell to him that we've got two Priority-1s.

As I get to the top level I see an unconscious crispy critter, a fireman, and another construction worker awaiting my arrival. It looks like his entire left foot has been blown off. Like his shoe exploded. I can see that his arm and upper chest were severely burned as the fireman removes his clothes. This was the first guy to grab onto the lines.

Note to self: don't ever grab power lines, *ever!*

We have to ABC this guy right here. I have to get him breathing. And, with any electrical injury, you have a good chance of the heart being screwed up. Remember, it's an electrical machine.

I crack open the Airway bag pull out the laryngoscope, I intubate the guy, start the BVM and get him breathing. This all goes so quickly because there's no resistance.

I feel for a pulse, and right now it's strong. So I continue to breathe for him while we get him strapped to the backboard. Then we all work together to hand him down. And it's just like moving a couch because there's no movement of his body when he's strapped in.

Ernie's patient is coding. He's a little older than my patient, and the electrocution seems to have affected his heart. I get my patient loaded into the unit.

Ernie is kind of on his own because I have to stay with my patient. He could crash at any moment. The electricity entered his right arm and exited his left foot. That means the arc of electricity went all the way through him.

Electricity always finds the path of least resistance. When my patient started getting zapped, his partner tried to pry him free. But, conductivity being what it is, the arc of electricity—as high as 30,000 volts in some cases—continued on through the good samaritan.

Ernie's patient took the electricity in through his left arm, across his chest, and out through his right arm. He looked like a wizard who had just shot out bolts of lightning from his toasted hands. And since the electrical current went directly across his chest that's probably why his heart is a quivering mess right now.

I heard Ernie saying something about a code, so I sent one of the firemen with the drug box and the monitor. Not more than 30 seconds later another ambulance shows up and it's my supervisor, Don. I send him in the direction of Ernie, informing him that his patient is crashing as we speak.

They grab their Airway bag and *Lifepack-10*, and haul ass to the scaffolding of death. And now it's starting to rain pretty hard, and around suspicious power lines that's never a good thing. What were they thinking?

I have to get going because my guy is in bad shape. Don's partner jumps in the unit with me and a fireman gets behind the wheel. I'm still breathing for the guy and I hand it off to the other paramedic and slap on the fast-patches.

Looking at the monitor I see a Sinus Tachycardia —fast heart beat, close to 120 bpm—with multi-focal PVCs (Pre-mature Ventricular Contractions). The *multi-focal* means that the heart is receiving electricity from different directions. And it lets us know that the heart did sustain damage from the electrical shock.

I call Medical Control and advise them of the situation. We're still a good 20 minutes from the hospital, so I'm just trying to keep my guy's heart beating. They tell us to administer some lidocaine which I do through an IV that I've recently started. That's to try to get rid of the PVCs.

The lidocaine seems to help his cardiac rhythm a bit. And now we just transport him as fast as we can.

Just a few minutes after we get him to the hospital, we notice Ernie coming in with his patient. He is in cardiac arrest, so we help him with the transfer into the emergency room.

They stabilize my patient right away. Ernie's patient is a clinical save—bringing him back to life—in the emergency room. But I believe that my patient, the first guy, he ended up losing both of his hands, and both of his legs below the knee. I guess the electrical current couldn't make up its mind exactly which direction to go in before it exited his left foot. So he was left a quadruple amputee.

Ernie's patient ended up losing both hands.

And of course, everybody in the world got sued on this one. The case took years to settle, and during the time between the incident and the settlement, one of the patients died due to complications from the original shock. He passed away in the burn unit while his family stood outside a glass window powerless to help him.

But they were alive when they left our ambulances. Nobody dies in an ambulance. Everything after that is between them and God . . . or their HMO.

23
DOUBLE-BARRELED
MOTHER'S DAY

May 10th
Sunday, 7:21 am . . .

"Springfield Dispatch to Metro-EMS . . . medical call. Twenty-ninth and Maiden Lane. Possible suicide."

I hear my radio squawking as I use an endotracheal tube stylette—a flexible tube, sealed in plastic coating, used to form the endotracheal tube for insertion—to fish candy out of the snack machine at St. Johns. I wouldn't normally be apart of such petty thievery, but the machine stole my last dollar and I have to draw the line somewhere.

We end up here at the hospitals, most mornings, because we get the majority of our transfers in the early hours of the day.

Just about the time I've got my *Peanut M&Ms* on their way to freedom, I hear, **"Medic-thirteen . . . what's your location?"**

"Medic-twenty-three," I answer, " . . . we're right around the corner from that call."

My supervisor then informs dispatch, **"Metro-EMS to Springfield Dispatch . . . Metro-three is en route."**

Ernie and I head out, my stomach grumbling something fierce. Score one for the vending machine.

When we arrive on the scene the police are already there. We're at a local motel that usually caters to families who have a loved one in the hospital. We make our way to the biggest accumulation of cops and notice that nobody seems to be in much of a hurry to do anything.

We carry the monitor and Airway bag, just in case. Right as we walk into the room we see a man sitting on a couch that backs against the right side wall of the motel room. He's sitting there, surrounded by cops as if he's being interviewed. But as we get closer we realize that his problems are bigger than a police interrogation.

His head is leaning forward, his chin touching his chest.

There is blood and saliva pouring from his mouth, and it's mixed together and coagulated. Try and imagine a red, frozen waterfall going from his mouth to his chest.

In the man's left hand is a crumpled photograph. It's old, the colors faded almost to black and white, the image grainy and devoid of any life. Oh, I almost forgot . . . there is a giant gaping hole in the back of his head with a big red spray pattern of blood and brains and hair on the wall behind the couch.

The way the blood is in a V-shape, I think back to my firefighter training. The V always points to the source. "Hey, Ernie," I say as I cross my arms like I'm looking at a piece of abstract artwork, " . . . it's pointing right at him."

Ernie shrugs and holds up the monitor as if to ask if it's really necessary to hook the leads up.

I nod, "Yeah, Ernie . . . hook him up."

We hook the leads up to his left ankle, his left arm, and the right side of his neck. "I'm fairly confident that we won't get any readings. And sure enough he's asystolic—flat line. We run the two strips off, say our goodbyes, and head out.

It's lunch time, and *Cici's Pizza* has a $3.99 *all-you-can-eat* buffet. It's a little out of our price range, but we just got paid yesterday. Besides, we love it when they see Ernie coming because they all collectively cringe and start whispering out the side of their mouths. Ernie can substantially affect a restaurant's bottom line.

32 minutes later . . .

"Springfield Dispatch to Metro-EMS . . . medical call. Six-fifteen St. Louis."

Ernie is just into his 4th plate of pizza and I just got done watching a 10-year-old kid vomit an entire pizza. As in . . . 12 chewed-up, finely liquefied slices, pepperonis and all. It was like a scene out of the *Exorcist*. Just when I thought he'd stop, another pitcher of chum comes spewing out. At one point Ernie stopped eating and said, "Is he kidding?"

"Let's take this call before we have to haul this kid," I say as I stand. "Besides, you're on a diet, anyway."

I grab my radio, "Medic-thirteen to Medic-twenty-three . . . our unit is pretty close to that location if you want us to take it."

"*Medic-twenty-three to Medic-thirteen,*" Don comes back, and I can hear sirens blaring in the background, " . . . *I'm already en route. You can meet us there. We're unsure what's going on at this time.*"

Ernie and I hit the ambulance and within four minutes we're pulling up to the curb of this old house. Just as we get the engine shut off I see our supervisor's unit skid to a stop in front of us. I glance at the house and notice that the front door is wide open, and that the place is eerily dark. There aren't any police officers, nor any first responders.

We're almost never the first to arrive on a scene.

I get out of the ambulance and walk over to Don, "Hey, are you sure this is the correct address?"

On the porch is a worn out old couch. The kind of thing I'd expect to see at the Tramp Camp.

Don lifts his radio up and asks, "Metro-EMS to Springfield Dispatch . . . can you give me the address for the Sixth Street medical call again? We're at Six-fifteen St. Louis?"

" . . . *Six-fifteen St. Louis, that is the correct address of the call,*" Dispatch replies.

Don shrugs as he gets out of his unit and we both stare at the rather creepy looking house. In the background we hear sirens approaching. The cavalry must be on their way.

I look at Don, "I'm not going in there until it's been secured."

This is about scene safety. We almost never arrive before police and fire. Not to an emergency call that is vague. And that is especially true if the call might be violent. And you always assume it's violent if you don't know any better. It might be grandma's just fallen in the tub. Or, grandma might be holding a butcher knife or a .38 special, thinking the neighbors are trying to kill her.

So, to avoid any unnecessary gunfire, we let the cops dash in and get into shootouts and exciting stuff like that. We don't carry guns.

Within minutes two police cars and a firetruck arrive on the scene. The cops clear the house for us to enter. They lead us to a back bedroom, telling us '*not to hurry*'. This place looks lived-in. Not so much dirty, but messy. There are clothes all over the place, and open dresser drawers, and the bed is unmade. Unkempt. To add to the aesthetic, imagine faded lime-green walls.

What we see is a man sitting on the bed, his body laying back, with his feet still on the floor . . . next to the double-barrel shotgun. And this guy looks 17 kinds of *dead* dead.

The room looked to be completely covered and sprayed with blood and brain matter, with bits of bone fragments and hair strewn throughout. It looked like somebody set off a head-bomb! Every square inch of the green walls, ceiling, and shaggy carpet floor were covered in death.

"That's two today!" Ernie says as he backs slowly out of the room. He didn't want to get dripped-on by the insides of this guy's head.

I delicately walk forward to hook up the leads. As I lean in I can smell alcohol. These kinds of things are usually preceded by a healthy dose of liquor. I hook the leads up under his shirt. The cables are extended all the way to the doorway where Ernie says, "Huh?"

"Huh, what?" I ask.

"He's got an agonal rhythm." That means there is just the faintest amount of electrical activity in his body. Some people call it a death rhythm, because it's so low. How this is possible I can't explain. He does-n't even have a head. Not one bit of it. I can't imagine a scenario where we could bring him back. And I'm fairly imaginative.

I grab one of the leads and pull it slightly so that it is no longer making contact with his chest. "Try it now, Ernie."

Ernie glances down at the monitor, "Oh . . . look at that . . . asystole." Asystole means, *no rhythm*. It means, *dead* dead.

"Run the strips," I say quietly.

Ernie pushes RECORD, and the monitor prints the record of the headless guy quickly. That's that. I wasted no time removing the other two leads. And as I stand to leave I see a huge, framed painting of Jesus Christ. And it looks like he's giving me the *glare*. You know, the accusative insinuating glare.

Those Jesus paintings, they're designed so that his holy eyes are always following you, wherever you go. Like those old Uncle Sam paintings where he's pointing at you no matter where you are in the room.

Well, in this bedroom, Jesus is watching everything, all the time. He's watching when you're sleeping and when you're putting on your clothes. When you bring some girl home, or have your playboys spread out across your bed while you try to fight open a bottle of hand lotion. Or when you pull the monitor lead off of a guy with no head that still reeks of bourbon so that you can officially document his death.

In those times, Jesus is watching.

But I don't really have a guilty conscience. If Jesus was better at doing his job, then I wouldn't have to answer calls like this so often.

I glance at Jesus, then around the room, at the lime-green and blood speckled walls, and I just shake my head. Then I turn back to Jesus, and he's got that *I'm so disappointed in you* look on his face. I just shrug and head out of the dripping bedroom.

Happy Mother's Day.

24
ORNERY
EXTRICATION

September 5th
Saturday, 7:40 pm . . .

"Springfield Dispatch to Metro-EMS . . . we have an injury accident at the intersection of Twelfth and Moffit Street. One of the vehicles is on its side. Unknown number of victims."

I answer the call within seconds, "Metro-EMS to Springfield Dispatch . . . Metro-three is responding from the West Station."

I turn to Ernie, "Hey, get your fat ass in gear!" But, as usual, he's more ready than I am. He races past me to the garage, and I take the rest of a Snicker's bar and shove it in my mouth as I follow him.

Moments later we're on the way. 12th street is only about five or so minutes away, but traffic is a little heavy tonight. It takes us just under eight minutes to get to the scene, and this is what we see: What looks like an old, maroon Dodge van is on it's side. The vehicle that seems to have collided with her was a blue Camaro.

They appear to have hit each other, driver's side to driver's side, coming from different directions. Ernie jumped out and checked the driver of the Camaro while a fireman and I jogged to the van.

As I get there the front windshield is smashed so that I could just reach in and start talking to the woman. She is laying on her side with her foot stuck between the passenger seat and the engine housing. I immediately go to hold in-line stabilization.

As I'm doing this, I'm trying to assess this woman. She's fat, smells like a cigarette factory, with mop hair and yellowed teeth. I don't want to say "white trash" but that's what is going through my head. There's this bright-eyed little cocker spaniel sitting next to her. And it looks like the dog might have been driving from the way they're positioned.

Trying to relax her, I smile and say, "You know, it isn't safe to let your dog drive in busy traffic like this."

"Oh, no," she says, "I'd never let him . . . " and then she gets it. "You're joking. That's funny." But she's not in a *funny* mood. She's scared to death.

Her eyes blinking anxiously, she says, "What's happening? Am . . . am I going to die?"

"No, no," I assure her. "You're going to be fine."

I need to calm her down so that I can get a C-collar on her. And since there's only just room for me in here, the fireman is getting the backboard ready so that we can slide it in and pull her out.

I'm trying to figure out how to get her foot untangled. It's like one of those MENSA puzzles.

I still haven't heard anything from Ernie. And out of nowhere I start getting punched in the back of the head. The first three or four shots take me by surprise because I can't register what's going on.

I can't turn to look because I have to maintain in-line stabilization in case this woman has spine injuries that we don't know about. There have been times where patients looked just fine, were placed on back-boards without the C-collar on, and then they got moved a fraction of an inch, and died right there on the spot.

It can happen.

So I continue to get punched in the back of the head while holding this lady's neck. And I start to yell, "Hey! Hello! Somebody is punching me! Is anybody paying attention over there? Seriously, I'm getting hit in the head and I'm trying to hold—"

And suddenly the punching stopped. Well, it stopped for me, anyway. Whoever was hitting me was now getting the fire stomped out of him by two burly firemen. And firemen are tough. These guys blow bubbles with beef jerky.

I get the C-collar put on, we get her on a back-board, all packaged-up. How I got her foot loose was to play a game of delicate seat adjustment, over and over. The seat was on a swivel so it just took the right combination of leverage.

I learned that, in a strange twist of events, her house is only just down the street. Her husband—the guy who started punching me in the head—had seen the accident and raced to her aid. Who knows what he was thinking? But now he's thinking it in the back of a squad car. He's going to spend the night in jail while his wife is in the hospital.

Their little dog, Taffy, was such a trooper through the whole affair. We brought him with us, letting him ride in the jump seat of the ambulance. He was really just the cutest little puppy in the world.

Unfortunately, the emergency room staff did not find Taffy as cute and cuddly as Ernie and I did, so we had to babysit the pup until animal control took him to be euthanized.

No. Just kidding.

We actually played with him for half an hour and then gave him to one of the family members who arrived at the hospital.

But just imagine if we had.

25
HEARTBREAK HOTEL

September 15th
Wednesday, 4:03 pm . . .

"Springfield Dispatch to Metro-EMS . . . medical call. Heart attack at Soul's Harbor. Fifteenth and Jackson."

"Metro-EMS to Springfield Dispatch . . . " my supervisor answers over the radio. His voice always sounds so hollow and distant through my radio, *" . . . Metro-eight is en route."*

Metro-8 is Ernie and I. We've spent the last half hour resupplying the unit. On the last call we took we had to crack the drug box and administer some Demerol. We had a young woman who took a nasty spill on a mountain bike.

I should explain the drug box. It basically works like this: The drug box looks like a large orange hard-plastic tackle box, which contains all of our emergency medications such as adrenaline (*epinephrine*), used to stimulate the heart during cardiac arrest, or for asthmatic patients, but in smaller dosages; Benadryl (*diphenhydramine*), for anaphylactic shock or allergic reactions; Dextrose, for diabetic emergencies; lidocaine, for stabilizing a patient's cardiac rhythm; nitro-glycerine, for chest pain and hypertension; Dopamine (*Hydroxytyramine*), which has a variety of uses like hypertension; Atropine, for heart rate and poisonings; and Narcan (*nalozone*), to reverse the effects of narcotics in relation to drug overdoses. There are several other drugs, but this is the basic list.

Then you have the box within a box, with its own specially numbered seal. And this is the *narcotics box*. Inside this box you'll find: Morphine Sulfate, for both medical and trauma pain management; Valium (*diazepam*), for seizures and anxiety; Demerol (*meperidine*), for pain management.

The narcotics box is sealed and set inside the drug box, which itself is sealed with a sticker and then a steel cable and padlock. And the keys to this padlock . . . they're sitting on my hip, clipped to my belt.

Well, by the time you've learned how to bring people back to life, you're resourceful enough to outwit a few small plastic seals.

The way it works is that any time you use any of the medications, you have to break a seal. Then, whatever amount you have left in the syringe after use, you must pour out in the presence of a nurse, or another paramedic. They will then sign your trip-sheet —a paper record of the call, from you're mileage to the treatments performed and medications used. There is supposed to be complete accountability for all medications used or discarded.

So what this means to Ernie and me is, after you use the drug box you drop it off at the station with the medic-in-charge, and he gives you a brand new one, with new seals that haven't been broken. And Ernie's big meaty hand just grabbed our new drug box. We jump into the unit, placing the drug box in the back, and then take off.

Now we're zooming! The way traffic is, it doesn't take us more than four and a half minutes to get there. As we drive up the street toward the shelter we see a building composed of red brick and wood panes. This building was constructed in the 1800's and looks like it. The downtown facility used to be an old retail shop of some kind.

Because of the poor lighting we opt to send the firefighters in first. In the event that anything shaky happens, which it sometimes does, they can be a buffer. Immediately upon our entry we find ourselves in an old lobby. This place smells aged and worn; musty, even. The air is stale and thick.

At the end of the lobby there is a locked door that we cannot pass without first going to a counter and dealing with a grim looking character who's missing most of his teeth. He's got dark, mean eyes and a chin you could use to open a can of tomatoes. He's the *check-in* guy. He's the man responsible for searching and guaranteeing that guests are not drunk, high, or introducing any paraphernalia into the facility. He's this place's version of St. Peter.

They have rather strict policies against alcohol and drug use, and this man looks like he's never taken a shot of anything in his life. He looks at us, squinting, like he's trying to see if we're going to pull a fast one. And for a moment he just stands there silent, like a human lie-detector. I bet he gives people this stare and they break down right then and there.

He clears his throat in such a way that I want to get a flu shot, and says, "Let me buzz you in." His voice is all scratchy and gruff. Lowering his shoulder he toggles some switch and the lobby door suddenly unlocks.

We enter into a very dark hallway, much darker than the lobby, where it was already hard to see much of anything. On the right side of the hallway there are boxes upon boxes of donated clothes and food items. But there is so little light that you can't make out much of anything.

One of the firemen quips, "All this donated stuff . . . you'd think there'd be some light bulbs."

The first area we reach is the Men's Dormitory. I expect we'll find our patient on the floor any moment. It looks like a World War II prisoner-of-war barracks. The bunk beds, made of nailed-together two-by-fours, cover every available square inch of the space. There's hardly enough room to walk down the middle. Blankets are hung on the sides of most beds as privacy screens, and to keep the draft at bay. There is a bone-chilling draft that routinely sweeps through this entire building and it's aching cold in the winter.

The check-in guy, who I later learn is a manager, urges us on, "He's up in the family sector."

We head down another hallway, passing the Women's Dormitory—a duplicate of the men's. We make our way into a narrow, dreadfully steep stairwell that climbs the red-bricked eastside wall.

After taking a couple of steps, hearing the groaning boards underneath me. I turn to Ernie, my face looking very concerned.

"Hey, you, ah . . . might want to let us handle this one, Ernie. You and these stairs," I shake my head, " . . . I'm not so sure."

He laughs, knowing that I'm just kidding with him about his weight. But seriously, he might actually fall through this time. These stairs seem like they incline at a 65 degree angle. This is the stair equivalent of a *Black Diamond* ski slope. I wager that many a hip and head have been broken after a missed step.

Like mountain climbers, we work our way up to the top and find ourselves in the Family Sector. Surprise, surprise, we find ourselves in another dimly lit hallway. There are several doors on each side of the hall, and behind each of these doors are rooms for entire families. These are the families that are either on a waiting list, or have been rejected by the Salvation Army. Apparently, they have some fairly stringent requirements for entry.

We negotiate the narrow hallway, noticing the peeling layers of old paint and plaster. The floor is hardwood stripped of any stain or coating. I feel like I'm in some Clint Eastwood movie and at any second a bunch of cowboys with six-guns are going to come running by shooting at each other.

We walk all the way to the end of the hallway, completely silent except for the static-laden sounds of chatter that squawk from our radios.

Ahead of us, at the threshold of one of the family rooms, is a fat woman wearing a nightgown with fluffy bits of material on the shoulders that might be hamsters she rolled over in her sleep. Her plump arm is flagging us down frantically . . . like we can't *see* her.

We get to the doorway and turn, and I see Robert Salter—the old guy who got stabbed in the Tramp Camp Riots—sitting in a green velvet chair. On the floor a few feet from his chair is a small half-range oven, and it's being used to heat the apartment. It's meant for hamburgers and hotdogs, but I suppose space heating will also do.

"Robert," the mean old check-in guy says, startling me. I didn't even know he was following us. Old toothless guys are creepy in ways I can't put into words. He points his wrinkled hand at Robert, " . . . you're not supposed to be up here. I'll let it go this time, but only because you're hurt." And after his reprimand he turns on his heels and disappears like a mist.

Like he was never there.

"How we doing, sir?" I ask as Ernie and I approach.

"My chest," he answers through worried eyes.

Robert is having severe chest pains so we get to work. Ernie drops the Airway bag, getting an oxygen bottle ready with a non-rebreather mask. I'm getting the monitor leads—small, sticky, circular pads—ready. It takes three pads, placed around the chest, in order to get a good EKG reading.

His EKG actually looks fine, but he says he's in immense pain, so he's quite anxious and fidgety. I glance at his stab wound and notice that it's starting to ulcerate—open, festering, unhealing wound. It looks like he pried the stitches off himself.

"Tell me where your pain is," I say to him. "And describe for me what your pain is on a scale of one-to-ten."

Instead of answering he just points to the right side of his chest, near his ribs. And I can't see anything there. No marks or bruising or apparent swelling.

"What *kind* of pain is it?" I ask carefully.

"A sharp, stabbing pain!" he answers quickly, his voice unsteady. I can tell he's scared.

I ask him if he's ever had pleurisy.

"What?!" he barks.

Pleurisy is inflammation of the *pleura*—the membrane that lines the thoracic cavity and folds in to cover the lungs. The inflamed membrane exudes varying quantities of fluid into the *pleural cavity*, between the two surfaces of the folded membrane.

I explain to him, "If you've ever had a lung infection, or lung problems, when your lungs heal you can get scar tissue. There are tons of nerves in your pleura, so it can be very painful."

I glance around, "In a dry environment like this, it can really flare up and give you grief."

"Well," he says, "I was a smoke-eater for twenty years." His reply, muffled through the translucent oxygen mask, lets me know he's starting to understand me. Smoke-eater, that's a reference to his firefighting career.

"I know, Robert," I said as I glance at the monitor. It still shows completely normal sinus rhythm. He doesn't appear to have any problems. But then, I'm not digging around inside his body.

I look at him, "Robert . . . you are not having a heart attack, okay."

"It hurts!," he snaps angrily. "It hurts and I can't stand it! I want a real doctor to take a look at me."

I scratch my head, glancing over at Ernie and the fireman. Well, once they request the ride, we *have* to give it to them. Alright, then. We help him to his feet and slowly walk him to the door, turning and heading toward the stairwell. The fireman sees a suitable chair that we can use to carry him down with, so he quickly snatches it up.

We're peering down the stairs from hell. I have to get my toes out over the edge before I can even see the other stairs.

We get him situated and begin to take him downward. Each and every step is a dice roll, and as we're about halfway down the stairs, I consider the predicament I find myself in. I'm below the chair that's holding crazy old Robert. Ernie is behind him, above the both of us. And I *know*, with a certainty that borders on omniscience, that if Ernie misses a step by so much as an inch . . . I'm a goner.

I'll be crushed in the avalanche of Robert and chair and Ernie. It will take rescue teams hours to dig out my corpse.

So, every step we take is a prayer, each footfall a chance of fate.

Luckily, we manage to make it down the stairs, and place Robert onto the gurney in a comfortable position. I then leave him with Ernie and the fireman so that I can jog ahead to the unit and call the hospital. I have to request orders for medication.

By the time Ernie and the fireman make it to the unit with Robert, I've already gotten the IV drip-set ready to go. I've been instructed to administer a *carpuject*—pre-filled syringe—of morphine sulfate to ease some of Robert's pain. I could use a little touch, myself, right now. But I digress.

I start an IV in Robert's left arm once we're safely inside the unit and he's fastened down. The fireman is driving, with Ernie back here beside the patient and me. And almost the instant the morphine hits his system, his pain subsides. He's a different man than he was 20 seconds ago.

Now it's quiet, again. Just like it was in that dark hallway. The loudest thing is the road beneath us.

"Didn't you guys have SCBA's in California?" I ask him. I'm referring to a Self-Contained Breathing Apparatus. Basically, I'm trying to strike up some light conversation with him to relieve the tension and anxiety that I still think he's feeling. Often, a pleasant conversation can do more than a box full of drugs.

Perception is reality. If you *think* you're doing better, you actually *get* better.

"Shit, boy," he says with a wry smile, "don't you know that the freshest air we could get was right inside our bunker coat collars."

I laughed. This is a different side of Robert. One I've never been allowed to see. Most likely, very few people have seen this facet of his personality. And I wonder why he lives the way he does. This is a man who has got a nice retirement. He has money. He's intelligent. He's got family that are living. He doesn't have to be a bum.

"Robert," I ask carefully, "is there any family that you want me to contact for you?"

He blinks a couple of times, considering my question and I notice that his personality is very familiar to me. When he's lucid and calm like this, he might as well be my supervisor, Don. If he said, "*Shooooo,*" right now I'd be sold. This guy is more than he appears to be. Greater than the sum of his parts.

He clears his throat. "They don't care about me, son," he says, swallowing very deliberately. "They just want my money. I'm a payday to them. And that *ain't* family."

I glance at the monitor again, making sure he's doing alright. Always reassess. ABC's. Even if they look alright, you constantly reassess. He's doing fine.

And as I look down at him, I have to ask, "Robert, why do you live like this? You've got money. You could live in a nice place, drive a fancy car. Eat warm food. Why this?"

He thought about my question for a long minute, his eyes dancing around, focusing on places I'll never be able to see. Images from his past that I can't possibly understand. And then his eyes find mine, "Too many pictures in my head. Too many demons."

And then he shrugs, "I couldn't be a part of that life, anymore. I had to walk away. Sometimes you *have* to walk away and never look back."

I nod, wondering if he is just me, 20 or 30 years from now. Am I seeing a glimpse of what I will become? Is this evolution? Is this humanity?

Or is this the lack of humanity?

And barely above a whisper, Robert echoes, "Too many demons. Too many demons."

I feel like bringing him home with me. Teaching him to like nice food and clean clothes and a soft bed, again. I want to clean him up and get him a nice suit. But the reality is that he's living the way he wants to. And who would I be to tell a man thirty years my elder what he does and doesn't want.

He's lost, and he chooses to stay lost.

I'm glad there's a Soul's Harbor for people like him. Several groups have tried to shut it down over the years, but they haven't succeeded yet. I hope they never do, because . . . where would all the people like Robert go?

26
Sticker Tag

June 16th
Wednesday, 11:23 am . . .

"Okay, Ernie," I whisper, "they just took their patient into the emergency room. They're going to be in there for at least ten minutes."

"I don't know," Ernie replies nervously, his eyes glancing around.

Right now we're huddled together around the corner from the emergency room entrance of St. John's Hospital. What we've been scheming about for the last couple hours is our full-on assault against Willard Country Ambulance Service.

As the designated PR guy for this week, I am armed with a full box of Metro-EMS stickers that we had leftover from a dog-and-pony show that we had at Lincoln Park Mall last weekend. The plan is to strategically place these stickers on all of the ambulances, blanketing the entire area.

We've already hit four of their ten ambulances this morning in a twilight attack. And now, after all of our early success, Ernie's getting a little shaky in the knees, worried about losing his part-time job with Willard County.

"They'll think I'm a spy," he tells me.

"You *are* a spy, Ernie. And you're doing the right thing." I slap him on the shoulder, "Come on, Buddy . . . let's do this!"

He still looks uneasy.

"War is ugly, my friend," I say to him. "But it's necessary."

The battle has escalated. As it turns out, they've been stealing more of our non-emergency transfers, hiding behind this bullcrap court ruling. It's gotten so bad that our board of directors is considering cutting one of the crews to part-time status.

And I remind Ernie of this in no uncertain terms.

"We're sending a message to these bastards that there's no place they can hide. We'll always be watching, waiting, and listening."

Last week we listened in on a scanner as one of the nursing homes—where I teach free CPR classes and give out sugar-free candy—called Willard County Ambulance Service non-emergency to a chest pain, which is *always* an emergency call. They knew that if they called 911, like they're supposed to, they would get sent our ambulance service. But Willard County is cheaper. They were just trying to save a couple of bucks, like it's even their money. We have been betrayed by this nursing home, and so have their patients.

Anyway, we're in the trenches now. Blood has been shed.

"We may have gone too far with that helicopter, Danny," Ernie says as his eyes dart suspiciously around. He's talking about a LifeFlight helicopter that we hit earlier. We got them good, stickers all over the inside of their cockpit.

I point to him, "That's what they get for fraternizing with the enemy. The friend of my enemy is my enemy, too!"

I nod. He nods. And we both take off across the parking lot, our eyes focused on the target—a blue and white striped ambulance with Willard County written all over it. We use several other ambulances and cars for cover as we make our approach. We're like super-ninjas, kind of. And I see that we've found Willard County Unit-12.

And she's a dandy.

I quickly slap a sticker on the back doors, right next to their emblem. The moment they reach to open the door, Metro-EMS will be staring them right in the face. That eerie sensation of being watched will creep slowly down their spines, wondering if we're still out here. They'll lose sleep. Their appetites will suffer. Paranoia, even.

I loud whisper to Ernie, "Now, do your part!"

He's got on latex gloves, opening a jar and scooping out a large gob of petroleum jelly. He waddles around to the front, driver's side door while I watch for unfriendlies. He then slimes the entire gob—and not a small amount, mind you—under the door handle. From 10 feet away I can actually hear it being slapped on. I'm hearing the same kind of sounds that you might be privy to during an enema. It's three kinds of disgusting.

He glances back at me and I give him the nod. And right before we can effect our escape a nurse walks past the front of the ambulance and turns, stopping dead in her tracks. She's just a few steps away from Ernie.

We're so busted.

Her eyes go from Ernie, to me, to the ambulance, back to Ernie, to his gloved hands, and then she squints.

"What are you doing?" the nurse asks as Ernie cowers, turning beet red.

And then I notice that we've been saved by the Gods. This inquisitive nurse, it's Megan! The *hot-tub-late-night-nurse-who-likes-threesomes* Megan. It looks like she had just come out for a smoke break. Ernie is uncomfortable enough around women, but when you add in the anxiety of being caught in the act of sabotage . . . he's nearly in a state of catatonic shock.

I walk slowly past Ernie, my movements calm and collected. I raise my index finger to my lips, saying, "Shhhhhhh." And then I whisper, "You never saw us. This never happened. We were *never* here."

And she smiles at me, laughing as she cocks her head to the side.

I wave for Ernie to head back to better cover, and once he's safely outside of earshot I whisper, "Call me."

She blows me a kiss and I turn and run with Ernie.

Ernie is still shaking, almost a quiver, as we scurry off across the parking lot. "We're done, Danny. That's the last one!"

"Done!" I say incredulously. "We're nowhere close to done. We're only halfway there." I shake my head as we get to the corner that gives us the best cover and concealment. "No, no, my friend. We've gone too far to turn back, now."

And before he can protest, I add, "Come on . . . we'll get some custard before we hit the other five units."

With a guy like Ernie, that's just about all it takes to secure his loyalty. We might eventually be referred to as insurgents for all of our shenanigans, but remember . . . one man's insurgent is another man's freedom fighter.

27
COWBOY UP!

June 25th
Friday Night . . .

I'm at the rodeo, working an extra shift with Brian—
the part time paramedic, part time dry-ice bomber.
Here's the basic layout: there are a bunch of rednecks
in bleachers circling a dusty arena where animals are
being tortured alongside a bunch of cowboys. There
isn't a single full set of teeth, nor a high school dip-
loma in the entire crowd.

This is a regular Saturday event. Brian and I are
parked at the far end of the arena so we can see all of
the action. And pretty much every five minutes somebody is getting hurt. But the thing with cowboys is,
they all want to shake it off. None of them want any
medical care because they want the injuries and scars.
They wear them like a badge of courage and honor. I
get it. It's stupid. But I get it.

We're eating nachos, drinking sodas, just hanging
around waiting for something so horrible that they
can't shake it off. Luckily for us, these kinds of accidents happen at least once per rodeo.

I'm finishing up a soda while Brian tells me about a girl he's dating as we watch another cowboy go down. They're doing bull riding right now. Brian's tale drags on, and right at the point in the story where he explains to me that his girlfriend is *not* a whore, this enormous bull rolls over the cowboy. It then precedes to have its way with the cowboy, hoofs and horns and everything. But, you know, this happens all the time.

We laugh as the clowns run out there to scoop him up, but they don't seem as enthusiastic as usual. In fact, the first clown to hit the scene starts raising his hands, flagging us over. Brian and I jump up, and run out there with a Trauma pack and the Airway bag. They've, of course, already corralled the bull. See, I'm not stepping one foot on that red dirt unless that big bastard is locked up.

And that's not about being scared, it's about scene safety. We can't save anyone if we're getting chased by wild animals. So Brian and I get there after the bull is safely gone and the first thing I notice is the cowboy, unconscious, laying on his back.

There are hoof prints on his head and chest. There's blood everywhere. And the guy doesn't look like he's even breathing. I immediately hold in-line stabilization, sending Brian back to get the backboard and the gurney. I'm establishing a secure airway because he's got blood coming out of his mouth. I intubate him, get the C-collar on, towel rolls beside his head, and get him taped and fastened onto the backboard.

Brian's handling the BVM for me while I cut off the cowboy's shirt and get the monitor patches on him. He's got a good pulse so we don't need the fast-patches yet.

All of this is before safety turtle-shells—protective safety vest designed for rodeos specifically—made their appearance on the competitive rodeo scene. Because of the lack of protection he's got several ribs broken. As I listen to him through a stethoscope I hear a distinct wheezing sound, as if air is being bled from a tire, and I know what that means.

He's got a sucking chest wound.

And that is problematic. Right away I cover the area on his right side where the frothy, bubbly blood is fizzing to the surface. I'm limited in what I can do with only one hand.

I have Brian cover the wound with his gloved hand, while I try to prepare a makeshift one-way valve—which is little more than a silicon glove taped down on 3 of 4 sides. That will allow oxygen and blood to escape, but prevent either from falling back into the wound.

We have to load and go. You might think, 'hey, what's the worst that can happen?' One of the complications can be that the lung is punctured and that it eventually collapses. He would then only have one other lung to oxygenate his cells.

The other complication could be that as the air collects in the lung cavity, it starts to exert pressure on the *mediastinum*—a division of the thoracic cavity that contains the heart, thymus gland, portions of the eso-phagus and trachea, and other structures.

As the pressure builds and gets exerted on the mediastinum it will push the heart and trachea away from the expanding lung cavity. This deviation impedes the function of all of the vital organs. That means that I have to really stay on top of an injury of this nature.

We race him back to the unit, get him loaded-up, and a volunteer firefighter appears. We get him behind the wheel so that Brian and I can work together on the patient.

Once inside the ambulance I get an IV started. We head out through the parking lot of the rodeo and we start to hear this thumping sound. The ride suddenly becomes very bumpy. Son of a bitch, we've got a flat!

The firefighter brings the unit to a stop and jumps out to check it. He yells, "We have a huge rock stuck between the two dually tires!"

It's not a flat, so that's good. But we have a patient with a *pneumothorax*—sucking chest wound—and that injury is slowly turning into a *hemothorax*—the chest cavity is filling with blood in place of air. And it might as well be a flat tire because we aren't going anywhere.

The cowboy has to get to a hospital as soon as pos-sible. Because of the ambulance being undrivable I go ahead and jump on the radio, "Springfield Dispatch this is Metro-eight . . . please dispatch LifeFlight immediately to the following location: Highway forty-four and County Line Road."

"Springfield Dispatch to Metro-eight . . . we copy. LifeFlight is en route."

Within two or three minutes LifeFlight calls us on their frequency asking me questions about the accident. I let them know that we were doing a stand-by at the rodeo, as well as all pertinent information.

And there's a system for this communication. The order is first and foremost, the *chief complaint:*

The patient is unconscious. He has a sucking chest wound or pneumothorax turned hemothorax on the right side. He has a head injury. He has a weak and thready pulse.

Then we call them about the *treatments* we have performed:

The patient is fully immobilized, C-collar, towel rolls, backboard. We have the patient intubated and respirations assisted. We have a one-way valve on the sucking chest wound. We have bilateral IVs hooked-up, pushing Lactated Ringer's. We don't seem to have any deviation of the trachea . . . yet.

"We're almost in the area. We think we've located your LZ. We'll see you shortly."

Less than a minute later I'm watching the helicopter land and we're racing across the parking lot with the unconscious cowboy. As we load him up I'm explaining everything I just explained to the flight nurse.

And then he disappears off into the sky. We were going to return to the rodeo but it seems like they've lost the heart to continue. Turns out, if one guy *almost* dies, they'll just call the whole thing off. Cowboys.

Brian and I get into the unit and head toward the hospital to check on the cowboy. What else do we have to do? Oh, yeah . . . we have this huge freakin' boulder in between our dually tires. So we're not going anywhere. Problems like this can be solved by our man The Chuck.

"Call The Chuck," I instruct. "He will help us."

And The Chuck was called.

And 18 minutes later he's looking at me like I'm completely inept, saying, "What'd you do to this one, Danny?"

"I didn't—" I try to answer.

"I guess we won't be haulin' this one like we did the last two, eh?" The Chuck says between cackles. He laughs like a coyote. Like a hungry maniacal animal.

But magically, and with a prowess I never thought possible in a wrecker driver, The Chuck has us back on the road in less than an hour.

The Chuck is wise.

28
DOG DAY

July 2nd
Friday, 7:31 am . . .

The most hectic day I ever had started the second that Ernie and I walked into the west station. The off-going crew hands us their radios before the door even closes behind us.

The crew chief—Richard—hands me the drug key, glancing at his watch, "They just called in an MVA and we're . . . off duty."

"We'd have taken it," his partner Brian adds, "but I've got a dentist's appointment."

"Yeah, yeah," Richard says, " . . . and I've got to drive him to the doctor."

"Dentist," Brian corrects.

"Right. That's what I said. Dentist." And then they both pass us and walk out the door.

Ernie smiles, shrugging as he takes off toward the unit. I go around and make sure the station is locked up and that the phones are correctly forwarding to the main station.

"Metro-EMS to Springfield Dispatch . . . Metro-eight is en route. Please make sure that Rural Fire is en route."

It's dark, pissing down rain, and the cloud cover is so dense that it could be nighttime if you didn't know any better. We're on our way to a motor vehicle accident at exit 17 off of Highway 44. People can't drive in this kind of weather. Cars are creeping here and there, lots of brake lights and sudden swerves. It takes us just under 10 minutes to arrive.

When we pull up the firemen are there holding in-line stabilization. The story is this: An elderly woman tried to make an exit off of the highway, but there was apparently some indecision on her part as to whether or not this was the exit she really intended. She lost control of the vehicle trying to pull back onto the highway, and commenced to collide with several white pole barriers on her way to a stop out in the grass.

She's quite shaken-up and scared, but most likely her injuries aren't life threatening.

We still take all precautions—C-collars, towel rolls, backboard, warm blanket. One of her wrists may be fractured, it's hard to tell at this point. But otherwise she's fine. We got her loaded up and I put a splint on her wrist, just to be safe.

Within minutes we were transporting her to the Medical Control Hospital.

Along the way I'm trying to comfort her, making small pleasant conversation. At one point she looks up to me with her light brown eyes and smiles, "You look just like my son."

"Well, thank you," I reply. What else could I say?

And then her face shrivels a bit, her eyes narrowing, "He's a real piece of work," she starts. Then she goes on and on about how he dropped out of school, married a slob, doesn't call enough, and that he has a horrible job selling insurance.

In a situation like this you just nod and smile until you can drop her off at the hospital. There, nurses and doctors will take the place of her other family members as she blames them for her family's suffocated and failed ambitions.

Ernie and I make pretty good time, despite the pounding rain, and within 20 or 25 minutes we've dropped off the woman, listened to some gossip about the nurses, and left. We have to get back to the station and resupply, even though we hardly used anything on the call. You always resupply when you can because you never know when the calls will start coming in, back-to-back.

And, luck as it is, we get another call when we're about 100 yards from the station.

8:43 am . . .

"Springfield Dispatch to Metro-EMS . . . medical call. FM three-thirty. Caller reports chest pain."

"Metro-eight is en route," Ernie replies.

This call is in the middle of nowhere. Anytime you hear the address as anything with FM—Farm-to-Market roads—you know you're going to the boonies. People will have very few teeth and plenty of ghost stories, and they'll all look alike, I just know it. Brothers and sisters get married in these parts.

It's raining so hard its coming down sideways and we can't see farther than 20 feet past the windshield. During the drive we get lost at least three times, and we finally have to call the Rural Fire guys and let them give us directions. We eventually arrive, after a profuse amount of profanity and U-turning.

As we pull up Ernie says, "You ever see *Texas Chainsaw Massacre*?"

"No shit," I say, looking at the dilapidated farm house. There just have to be bodies buried in the wet mud, or under the creaky floorboards of this place.

We bring the drug box, the Airway pack, and the cardiac monitor. There were already three firefighters on the scene, so they met us at the front door.

"Did you guys see any axes?" I ask.

"Huh?" one of the firemen replies as we all try to estimate when this place is going to collapse on our heads.

And the story is this: There is a 65-year-old man inside with a history of heart complications. He's had a bypass within the last five years. When we get inside I notice that the firemen have already got the patient breathing oxygen.

This is technically Ernie's patient. What we do is swap every call so that we don't burn out. That only works when both members are paramedics. If one of us was an EMT we'd have to let any advanced life support treatments be handled by the paramedic.

So on this one I'm just helping out, hooking the patient up to the cardiac monitor while Ernie interviews him. I'm getting the vitals, he's getting the history. The man claims to have *"crushing chest pains."*

Ernie gives him some baby aspirin and a nitro-glycerin patch—nitro glycerin ointment that we squirt onto a patch and stick on his skin.

By the time we're done with the basic patient treatment, the firemen, still wearing their street clothes, bring in the gurney and we get the man as comfortable as possible. There's a few ogling family members that make me wish I had a gun on me. I don't know if they're interested in our treatment, their grandfather, or if they're hungry for human flesh.

Since there's no immediate emergency with the patient I elect to drive the unit. We get the man out, loaded into the back, and I give the house one last glance. You know how houses can kind of have their own personality? Well, this was one of *those* kind of houses.

Chop, chop, then!

It takes us forever to get to the hospital. This is the time before everybody had GPS systems in their units. Now you could be stuck in the middle of Bosnia and make your way out without incident. But back then we used a combination of maps, cell phones, and cursing.

We arrive at the hospital and learn that our patient has already got a room in the Cardiac Care Unit waiting for him. We get our paperwork finished and head back to the west station. I've got designs on a microwave hamburger.

When we get back we give the unit a thorough cleansing, washing off the mud and rocks and pure evil that were stuck to just about every surface. There's brown and grey muck everywhere.

"Hey Ernie, you want to—"

And before the words can get all the way out of my mouth we get the call.

_12:17 pm . . ._

"*Metro-one to Metro-eight . . . patient transfer. Eighteen twenty-five Markwardt to St. John's Radiation Oncology.*"

"Metro-eight en route," I say before lowering my radio. I yell through the bathroom door at Ernie, "Let's roll, partner. We've got to beat Willard County or they'll be stealing *these* transfers, too."

Less than a minute later we are slamming the doors on our ambulance; Ernie grabbing his clipboard, me wondering how he finished up in the bathroom so quickly.

The trip takes us about 15 minutes, due to bad traffic and horrible weather conditions. We take the gurney and head into the living room of an elderly couple that live in a nice home with porcelain animals everywhere. Seriously, there were bears and horses and puppies and turtles. And I crap you not, I even saw a porcelain trailer. A double-wide, I believe.

The man's wife is very polite and she explains that her husband has an appointment, the third this week.

The story is this: The patient has lung cancer, and he's on an oxygen concentrator—pulls moisture and contaminates out of the air. This is a rudimentary, terribly simple procedure. All we do is put him on our oxygen and get him transferred.

But this guy is a little paranoid. So it takes us a while to persuade him that our oxygen is just as good as his. Finally he acquiesces, allowing us to unplug the end of his nasal cannula from his machine and quickly into our oxygen bottle. We've done it a zillion times, so it's really nothing.

Strangely, he's wearing a hospital gown, even though he's at his own home. As he moves I notice that he's still got the markings from the hospital on his chest. There are black dots, dashes, and a plus sign here and there. Those are the targets for his radiation therapy, letting the doctors know where to nuke him. The gown makes sense if he's getting nuked every other day.

We get him loaded into the back of the unit and set off for Radiation Oncology, which is just a satellite building near St. John's.

While we are driving, the old guy tells Ernie that he looks like one of his grandsons. And when I hear that I start to giggle.

"What's funny about that?" Ernie loud whispers.

"Nothing, Ernie. Nothing at all."

We deliver him to the Radiation Oncology department and set sail for the west station.

2:11 pm . . .

"Medic-23 to Medic-13 . . . you're patient's ready to go back home from Oncology."

Back in the unit we go. We head to St. John's and meet our elderly friend with lung cancer who thinks that Ernie is his grandson. We get him comfortable in the unit and transport him back to his home at 1825 Markwardt, and into the loving arms of his wife.

Ernie shakes her hand and smiles, but she gives him a suspicious glare. I guess he doesn't remind her of their grandson at all. Ernie looks at me dumbfounded.

"It's like looking at the clouds, Ernie. You see rabbits, I see prostitutes."

He scratches his chin as we're leaving. As we walk out we notice the sun shining for the first time in the last several hours. And it's quite warm.

3:40 pm . . .

"Springfield Dispatch to Metro-EMS . . . ALS intercept with Willard County Ambulance. They have a drowning patient."

I hear Medic-23 on the radio volunteering Ernie and I so we get up from the recliners in the day room and head to the unit. An ALS—Advanced Life Support—intercept means that the Willard County Ambulance guys are too far away from the hospital and they only have EMTs in their unit. See, we have a mutual aid agreement with them that says that anytime either of us need support, we'll help.

The turf war always ends the second a patient is involved. It's still about keeping people alive.

This is Ernie's patient, again, and as I'm driving I say to him, "I guess this will work out alright since you already know where everything in their unit is stored."

He brushes it off with, "I just use them for practice."

We meet the Willard County Ambulance EMTs at Highway 71. They pull over and we do a U-turn, pulling up directly behind them. As we get out we grab all of our gear—drug box, Airway bag, cardiac monitor—just in case they don't have theirs. You never know.

We both go to the back door of their ambulance and the first thing we see as the door swings open is a 7-year-old girl in her bathing suit strapped to a backboard. We quickly step up inside the ambulance to get closer.

She must have been at a swimming hole or something. One of the EMTs is breathing for her with the BVM. His eyes are wide and concerned, giving us the *help me* glare.

Ernie moves up to her head with his Airway bag. He sizes up her endotracheal tube and within seconds he's got her intubated, handing the BVM back to the EMT, who is still sweating bullets.

By this time I have her on the cardiac monitor which is showing a Sinus Tachycardia. But a fast heart rate is normal for a small child. Kids have strong hearts. I prep her for an IV, and start it in her left arm.

The EMT kicks on the lights and sirens and we take off, leaving our ambulance on the side of the road.

We call back to our main station and have somebody go and pick-up our unit. And for the next several minutes Ernie and I sat in the back constantly reassessing this fragile little girl. When we're working on a kid we don't talk much. No time for joking around.

We make it to the hospital and drop her off to the emergency staff. The little girl was immediately taken up to the ICU—Intensive Care Unit—and we head out to the parking lot where Medic-23 delivers our ambulance to us.

"Thanks, Don," I tell him as he tosses me a candy-bar.

"You boys look busy," he says, slapping Ernie on the shoulder. "It's just one of those days when everybody's trying to die. What happened with the little girl?"

"Swimming hole," I say. "She aspirated water."

He shakes his head, "Can you imagine being seven and drowning? Cold and darkness suffocating you?"

"Not until just now, Don," I say to him. "Thanks for the visual."

He and his partner take off and the second we get inside our unit we hear the tones going off.

"Are you kidding?" I laugh.

But no.

They weren't kidding.

5:18 pm . . .

"Springfield Dispatch to Metro-EMS . . . thirty-one hundred Sunset Drive. Caller is home healthcare, asking for assistance with a patient."

That could mean just about anything. The patient could be coding, bleeding to death, floating around possessed by the Prince of Darkness. Anything! So we light 'em up and haul tail.

Over the next half hour we race to the house where we learn that a nurse was having real trouble getting one of her patients lifted out of a bathtub. It's difficult because patients, even live ones, feel like dead weight.

It turns out that the patient was fine and the nurse began apologizing the second we walk in the door. She says there was a mix-up between her and dispatch, and she thought she had made it sufficiently clear that it was a non-emergency call.

But, you know, wires cross.

We wave off the firemen, and I key-up, "Metro-eight to Springfield Dispatch . . . this will be a dry run. No transport. We're available."

"Copy that, Metro-eight."

Then we help her lift this short round woman out of her bathtub. It was like moving a walrus or a sea-cow from a tank at SeaWorld. Seriously, it even smelled like fish.

10:26 pm . . .

"Springfield Dispatch to Metro-EMS . . . medical call. Northwest corner of Eighteenth and Lone Elm. Asthma attack at the fiberglass plant."

"Metro-EMS to Springfield Dispatch . . . Metro-eight is en route," my supervisor says, offering our services.

To which Ernie replies, "Gee, I thought they'd never call."

"Don't jinx us, Ernie," I say as we step into the unit. We flip on the lights and the sirens, floor it, and within four minutes we're skidding to a stop in the Frontier Fiberglass parking lot. The fire captain is already on the scene and he meets us.

The story is this: A guy was working with some acetone and he was overcome by fumes. This instigated an asthmatic attack. Asthma is a very common, but confusing medical condition.

Basically, exposure to an inciting factor stimulates the release of chemicals from the immune system that cause spasmodic contraction of the smooth muscle surrounding the bronchi. This causes swelling and inflammation of the bronchial tubes, and excessive secretion of mucus. The inflamed, mucus-clogged airways act as a one-way valve—air is inspired but cannot be expired. The obstruction of airflow may resolve on its own, or with treatment.

This patient's going to be mine.

The first thing we do after the ABC's it to get him on oxygen. We then use an SVN-Nebulizer full of Albuterol Sulfate. It's a bronchodilator—which relaxes smooth muscle constriction and opens the airways. This is to open the bronchial pathways, making it easier for the alveoli to exchange oxygen and carbon dioxide. I then give him a shot of Benadryl.

He's conscious right now, but if he were to go unconscious we would have had to intubate him very quickly. Otherwise his trachea would swell shut and we'd be doing an emergency tracheotomy—cutting a hole in his throat to breathe. Fortunately for us that doesn't happen.

We monitor him closely as we get him packaged-up and loaded into the ambulance. Minutes later we are pulling in to the hospital parking lot. And wouldn't you know it, he turns to me, kind of tugging at my shirt, "You know, you look like that guy on TV."

"Which guy?" I ask.

"You know . . . that guy who sells cars off of Forty-four."

Oh. "Well, I'm not him. I don't sell cars."

"Right," he says. But judging from his narrow eyes I can tell he's not convinced.

12:47 am . . .

"Springfield Dispatch to Metro-EMS . . . motor vehicle accident at Fifteen-hundred Campbell Road. Patrol car involved."

Ernie and I are sitting in the day room preparing to watch a movie that we had rented a few days ago. We're sprawled back on the recliners, with bubbling sodas between us. And though we're determined to watch this tape before we have to return it, chances are, that isn't going to happen.

Medic-23 volunteers us for the call since we're closer, and as we hear his voice we both audibly sigh. More of a groan, really.

"Let's not keep them waiting," Ernie quips as we get up and head to the unit. I don't know how he stays so damned chipper all the time. He loves this stuff.

We roll out, lights and sirens blazing. If we can't relax, nobody else is going to either. Wake up Springfield! Somebody is dying.

We make our way to the scene and as we pull up we see two firetrucks—a pumper and a rescue/beer truck —but we don't see any crashed vehicle. We know it's around here somewhere. But where?

I get out and ask the captain, "What's going on?"

And the story is this, whispered to me all conspiratorially, "The guy's not hurt. Well, not physically. He thought he was on Twentieth Street, but he was actually on Fifteenth."

Uh-oh. Twentieth Street continues on past Campbell Road. But 15th dead ends. So, obviously you might have problems if you forgot where you were. Like some drunken idiot.

"Well, everything after that is a field," I say. "You'd have to be a real dipshit to forget where you were." I look around, "So . . . where is the car?"

The captain points out into the field. And sure enough, about 50 yards down the bank I see a flipped-over cop car. "Captain, you know the first rule of racing?"

"Yeah," he laughs, " . . . keep 'em on the rubber side." Then he points to the rescue truck, "The trooper is sitting in the truck." And I can tell that the captain is physically fighting the urge to laugh.

When I open the door to check out the trooper I notice it's Lieutenant Styles. This guy is a supreme douche bag. A month ago this asshole gave me a ticket on my way in to work. I told him I was being called in and was wearing my uniform, but that didn't seem to matter. I guess he'd never heard of professional courtesy.

And now the prick is my patient. Right now he's just holding a 4-by-4 bandage to his forehead. That's probably where all of the dumbass-goo leaks out of him.

"How you doing, officer?" I say, restraining my smile.

He instantly recognizes me, "I don't need no ambulance." And then he shakes his head, "I'm fine."

Fine.

"Good," he says, almost snorting as the muscles in his jaw tense.

Wonderful.

"If you don't want treatment then you'll need to sign this refusal form, sir," I say, fishing out the document.

He snatches it from my hand. I make sure he signs the refusal form. And once I have it safely in my pocket, I tell him, "That's alright. We'll just get some photographs for our records and be on our way."

It seems like the idea takes a few seconds to bounce around inside that prick-thick skull of his. And then it begins to enrage him. "Oh, I bet you love this. I bet this is the highlight of your day. You'll take a bunch of pictures and have a nice laugh."

Normally I would ignore these kind of petty jabs, but this dick had it coming. Especially after the day we've had.

"Yes, sir," I say with a smile, "we are. This will be the high point of our week. I'm going to have a big party and make hundreds of copies so that everyone can enjoy this moment forever. We'll be joking about this for years."

And then Ernie and I take a walk down the bank and spend an entire roll of film. Every click was a smile. Every flash in the darkness was another chuckle.

Karma is a bitch.

4:21 am . . .

"Springfield Dispatch to Metro-EMS . . . we have a burn at the Greyhound bus station."

Ernie and I roll out of our too-small beds at the sound of our supervisor's voice coming over the radio. I bet Don's having a good laugh tonight.

We get into the unit, light 'em up, and run emergency the whole way. Six minutes after I opened my eyes, I'm pulling up to the bus station.

The fire department is there, they just woke-up themselves. Their hair is crazier than Ernie's. The captain points over his shoulder, "It's a, uh," and then he just motions us past him, as he shakes his head.

Once we enter, the florescent lights making everything look like a bad commercial, we see one of the firefighters taking vital signs from a red woman.

Really red.

Cherry red.

And here's the story: This woman in her early 30s just came back from some kind of vacation where they hold you next to the sun for as long as it takes to turn your entire body red.

Seriously, I have to squint when I look at her. She looks like a fake person. A copy of a real person, spray painted red.

I turn to Ernie, "Well, pal . . . you're up."

The first thing he asks is, "Uh . . . do you *really* want to go to the hospital? For *this*?"

And she looks him dead in the eyes, her jaw tightening, "Absolutely."

So we all groan in unison as we turn and go to fetch the gurney. We lay her down and take her out to the unit. None of us say much in the back of the ambulance as we're driving to the hospital. There have been so many calls in the last 20 hours that I don't remember where we even started.

The only thing that brings a smile to my face is when she stares at me and says, "Hey, you know what . . . you look like my ex-boyfriend."

"Thank you," I answer tiredly.

"No, really, he was a complete dick," she said, almost spitting. "I *hate* him."

"Thank you," I reply. "He sounds like a great guy."

And Ernie, the pal that he is, he starts snorting, trying not to laugh outright. Choked laughter. Bridled hilarity.

What a long night.

We drive along in the silence, only the sounds of the road and the wind whistling by us.

Just then it starts to sprinkle again, the raindrops exploding into smaller beads of water when they hit the windows. "The rain is back," Ernie says to nobody in particular.

"It's always raining around here," I say to the darkness.

29
METHIN' AROUND

August 8th
Sunday, 5 am . . .

We're late into our shift and the phone starts ringing rapidly. Like the phone is in a hurry or something. We're at the main station trying to catch a cat nap, but with all the racket I can't keep my eyes closed. I notice my supervisor on the phone, doing a lot of nodding and *okay*ing and feet shuffling.

Ernie and I are being lazy bastards in the day room. He's spread out on the sofa, looking fatter than a bloated hippopotamus. I'm laid back on the recliner, seeing if I can get far enough back to touch my head to the floor. Some dick on TV is selling a plastic food cutter that apparently chops vegetables into pieces the size of hydrogen atoms.

And I realize that this call is probably coming our way. When we're at the main station we rotate calls. Three paramedic teams means we get every third call. And this is lucky number three.

Our supervisor has been milling around for hours because he has to log in all of the calls from the previous day. And he always sits at the kitchen table to do this. It's his ritual, kind of an unspoken quiet time that we try not to disturb. Don likes his kitchen time.

He hangs up the phone and calls to me, "Danny . . . Ernie, you guys awake?" He then walks in and hands me a piece of paper, "We have an SRT standby at Twenty-seventh and Iowa. Maintain radio silence. You'll stage at the intersection of Twenty-sixth Street. It's a possible haz-mat."

Ernie and I get up quickly. SRT is the police Special Response Team. Ernie's eyes get all wide and excited. This is like the holy grail of calls for him. So I practically have to run behind him to keep up on our way to the unit. In less than a minute, we're pulling out of the bay into the cloak of darkness.

It takes us just over 10 minutes to get to the scene because we aren't running emergency. As we pull up to the staging area at 26th and Iowa, I notice a firetruck and police car parked nose to nose, blocking the entire street.

All of the houses in the immediate area have been cleared of their inhabitants, and this boundary extends for a block in every direction. The area immediately around the target house is surrounded by the SRT guys. They're wearing all black combat fatigues, with machine guns and vests and helmets.

Really, they kind of look like Nazis.

The area that circles the Nazi controlled territory, around the target house, is blocked off and filled with policemen and their vehicles. Then there is a third ring beyond the policemen, where medical personnel and firemen are staged. Beyond us are the gawking public which we try to shoo away on a fairly routine basis, but it never works.

In the police ring there is a large, boxy transport vehicle that reminds me of a big ambulance, but with enough space for several Nazis and their machine guns.

Ernie and I have done SRT gigs before. They always take a long time, and end rather abruptly, like most of my relationships. I make my way over to a firefighter that I know and we shake hands.

Near us a police vehicle with a German Shepherd in the back. It's the K-9 unit. Just as I'm about to take a step in to see the pooch, this lady police officer barks at us to stay away from her dog. Like she owns it.

We back away, not answering her. We don't talk to cops if we don't have to. They're typically arrogant and treat us like we're second-class citizens. We're the dogs to them.

Ernie, the firefighter, and I stare past the layers of police activity and focus on the target house, a run-down place if I've ever seen one. If it collapsed into a dusty fog I wouldn't be surprised. If the ground opened up and swallowed it hole, I'd barely shrug.

"Shithole," Barry the firefighter says under his breath.

"Copy that," I agree.

"So what's the story, Barry?" Ernie asks quietly, as if we're not supposed to be talking.

The skinny of it is this: Some guy has his wife inside the house, held at gunpoint. He's very angry, probably suicidal, and has a propensity for drug abuse. Oh, yeah . . . and he's been taken downtown for beating his wife on more than one occasion.

This is the kind of guy you see on *Cops*, wearing a mean face, a stained wife-beater shirt, with most of his teeth missing from opening beer bottles with his mouth for decades, and his wife is in the other room crying, " . . . he only hits me 'cause he loves me."

In a nutshell, this guy is a scumbag puke.

But something about the call was still bothering me, "Hey, Barry, what . . . what was the haz-mat warning for?"

Haz-mat means hazardous materials—contaminants of a biological, radiological, or chemical nature. And my supervisor had specifically mentioned it.

He lowers his voice, "There may be a drug lab inside."

So, standing in ring three, the three of us peering past the tense police officers and their Nazi SRT guys, we reminisce a bit.

It wasn't too long ago that we had a standoff where a guy had been sexually assaulting his ex-wife all night long with a broken broom stick. Somehow she had wrestled away the gun he had been using to control her and managed to called 911.

SRT and what looked to be legions of local police officers had surrounded the house while she was on the inside, now holding the gun on her abusive husband. When they were done screaming at each other she forced him, at gunpoint, to run out the front door into the yard at a full sprint. She was hoping that the cops would unload on the guy and all of her troubles would be solved.

And shoot him they *did*, just not with bullets. They used non-lethal beanbags, much to her disappointment. As the bags made contact, he went ass over elbows to the ground, where he was knocked-out. These beanbags can be fired from a regular shotgun. The projectile expands after it leave the barrel, and when it hits it basically knocks the piss out of you, but doesn't break the skin.

Anyway, the guy got hit five or six times and thought he was dead. When we finally entered the scene and cut his clothes off he had enormous black welts all over his body. It looked horrible. We packaged him up like we would any other patient and got him to the hospital.

Along for the ride were two police officers that didn't appear to have any sense of humor at all. I remember that being a particularly long night.

Barry hands me a cup of coffee, "Hey, you remember the jackass who blew his brains out on the front porch?"

"Oh, yeah," I said.

Ernie nodded as he took a sip of scalding hot coffee. You could drop chunks of metal into this coffee and they would melt instantly. It's right at the boiling point of ferrous metals.

Trying not to burn the skin off our lips we talk about another SRT call where we had a man threatening suicide. I always thought that was a rather asinine threat to make to a bunch of guys who are pointing guns at your head. *'Back off or I'll blow my brains out.'* That kind of ultimatum would be met by disinterested shrugs and maybe some whispered taunting in Chicago.

Anyway, inside that particular house there were three family members being held hostage. The man was inside making all kinds of threats and requests for completely ridiculous junk. He didn't want a bus, he had to have a 'tour' bus. He wanted some ridiculous amount of money that all the banks in the world probably couldn't come up with. There was just no negotiating with the guy. The whole ordeal lasted longer than three hours. *Bo-ring.*

That's why they call it a standoff. Not like he was standing with his hand hovering over his Colt pistol while the cops were staring him down waiting to draw. Nothing like that. It was mostly cops sipping coffee while a Crisis Negotiator tried to explain why it may take some time to arrange a private, gold-plated, 747 with pink leather interior, on such short notice.

Well, without any warning, the guy walks out onto the front porch, gives the crowd one good look, and then raises his .357 revolver to his right temple. He then glares at one of the Nazis, laughs to himself, and pulls the trigger.

Pop!

Think of a thick spray of red and gray and bone white with a little black hair mixed in there. Now imagine all of that stuff painting the floor and window and wall of the front porch. This was like some cheesy B-movie. But it wasn't a movie. It was a guy named

Walter, turning his head and grey matter into a spectacle.

Our treatment was rather simple on him. We walked up, kneeled, and hooked-up the monitor leads so that we had a printout of the flat line. Even when a person is dead we need a legal record of it. They've been having us do that ever since *Mike the Headless Chicken* lived for 18 months after having his head chopped clean off by a farmer. Can you imagine?

So here we are now, a cup of coffee in our hands.

Barry turns to Ernie, "What about that chick who —"

Ka-booooom!

We all feel the explosion rattle deep in our chests. From a block away we see the front picture window of the target house explode, glass spraying in every direction like tiny flying razorblades. I believe the Nazis used a concussion grenade—also known as a flash bang —to surprise and subdue the man in the house. It surprised me enough to spill some coffee, so I figure anyone in the house has probably evacuated their bowels at this point.

Outside you could hear a pin drop, we're all so quiet. There was a bunch of shouting. And then it got quiet for a second . . .

Pop-pop-pop!

Three more shots echoed around us.

Then lots more shouting.

Two Nazis appear from the house carrying a woman who had been hog-tied. They quickly carted her past the first barrier, dropping her on her stomach in the second ring, where all of the police are waiting expectantly.

I hear our radios start to squawk, *"Springfield Dispatch to Metro units . . . Springfield police are signal-seven. They are requesting paramedics and firefighters at the squad cars."*

And just about the same moment that the calls come over the radio we see several police officers waving at us. Ernie and I bring the gurney and all of our gear and make our way toward the hog-tied female. When we get there she's laying on her back, her hands cuffed in front of her. She's conscious but woozy, as if she just got off of a carnival ride.

Ernie starts working on her, getting her immobilized on the backboard. She has glass cuts all over her body, so she must have been close to the window. While he's doing treatment on her, one of the police lieutenants asks me to come in and look at the other body. They don't say patient, they say *body*.

He tells me, "Don't touch *anything* except for where the monitor leads need to go." And since he's still salivating from the assault I don't give him any lip.

I have on two pairs of gloves, with just the Lifepak-10 monitor hanging over my shoulder. As soon as I get in I can smell the fetid coppery odor of blood mixed with sewage and strong solvents of some kind. Like cleaning chemicals, maybe.

As I kneel down I hear one of the Nazis yelling from somewhere deep in this dark house, " . . . a functional meth-lab!"

Methamphetamines are made by combining a bunch of poisonous and explosive chemicals in order to make an even more horrible compound. And your *chemists*, they're usually guys who didn't get past the 6th grade. They can't be trusted to cook a hot dog, but people inject their concoctions into their veins.

For reasons beyond my comprehension the floor in this house looks like dirt. No foundation. No carpet. Just packed clay. This entire place looks like the inside of some disgusting garage.

It's dark and moist in here. Everything is rusted and falling apart. As my eyes adjust I see a red plastic canister of gas in the far corner of the dining area. Umm . . . why?

There is a freaking chainsaw in the living room. *Who does that?* Is a chainsaw so important that you need it next to the table you eat off of? I don't know how anyone could live in an environment like this. I'm here 30 seconds and I feel my life ebbing away.

This awful, dilapidated house is in the middle of a sad rundown neighborhood. It's surrounded by Nazis and cops who don't care if the inhabitants live or die, in a town of people who take pains to avoid even driving in this general area.

There is no hope here.

None.

I'm wondering if the floor rotted away sometime between the late 1800s, when it was built, and now.

I steady myself over the body. This guy's got long greasy black hair, a dirty tank-top with a plaid shirt over it. He's got on dark blue Dickeys pants, muddy work boots, and three career ending gunshot wounds. No beanbags here.

One round in the stomach—adding to the stench.

One in the left lung cavity—guaranteeing he couldn't breathe.

And one just above his upper lip—the one that turned off the computer. Forever.

I carefully placed the leads on his chest—red on the lower left rib cage, black on his left shoulder, and white on his right shoulder. In order to announce someone dead you have to have a printout on at least two readings from the monitor's thermal printer. Those printouts show conclusively that this is not *Mike the Headless Assailant*, and they end up in our report later. We'll also attach a summary of the incident that lead to his death.

At some point, all of this stuff will end up as evidence in court. But for us, a patient is a patient. A body is a body.

Just another DRT.

Dead dead.

Ernie hollers that he's ready to go with the female patient, and since I don't even have a patient, I'm pretty much done. I remove the leads, get up quickly, and I'm on my way.

We load up into the unit and head to the hospital. After we drop the woman off to the emergency room staff we are made to exchange our clothes for scrubs while our stuff is specially laundered. Since we came into contact with hazardous materials at the scene, especially me, our stuff will have to be handled carefully.

And it makes me wonder how bad meth must really be for you if even your clothes need special treatment when they are exposed to the kinds of ingredients used to produce the drug.

We learned later that the woman was a part of the methamphetamine lab conspiracy. The rest of their family, with all of their slowly rotting teeth and black eyes, were sitting in the county jail pending drug charges.

I think back to that dead guy, the life sucked right out of him, often. I think about his house, which also appeared to have had all of the heat and life leeched from it. I realize that life can take it out of you, or you can choose to take it out on yourself.

This dead junkie, he probably had the time of his life, right up until it all went black. But remembering that house, who knows when that might have been. A guy like that, maybe he was looking for a quick way out. Maybe this was a protracted suicide? The Nazis, the bullets—perhaps that was all part of the plan. Instead of a western standoff, this could have been a premeditated suicide-by-cop.

But I don't have the time to ponder all of that. I've got more pressing issues. Ernie and I have to get some breakfast.

30
MONEY HUNGRY

September, 17th
Sunday, 11:47 am...

We're just sitting around on a quiet Sunday morning. The golden fingers of sunlight are just starting to fall down onto the carpet after having spent the last couple of hours sliding along our walls.

We hear the front door open, up near the reception area, and then people start calling out, "Is there anybody here?"

"Help!" a woman's voice cries out.

Tim jogs his squirrelly tail by us to the front while Don walks behind him, calm and collected as always. I follow behind Don, not making any effort to run. We don't run. Unless alien tripods are stomping their way down Main Street, we're not going to even jog.

This family, dressed in their Sunday's best, are pulling a major freak-out. They're talking excitedly about something outside. You'd think the world was ending the way they're going on and on. A young man in his mid-20s takes Tim by the arm and half drags him as he points across the street to the parking garage.

Don is being his normal relaxed self, trying to keep everyone from going crazy.

Tim heads out with the young man as Don turns to me and nods. I go and fetch the equipment—Airway bag and monitor—and follow them out. See, you can't do anything without your medical equipment. I know this. Don knows this. Heck, the frightened family may even know this. But it is apparently lost on Tim during the excitement of the moment.

As I get outside I notice that they're all heading straight to the condemned parking garage across the street from the station. Coincidentally, that is the same parking structure where we did our dry-ice terrorist attacks some time ago. People still giggle about that in the station.

I make my way across the street and climb over a chain as I enter into the darkness. It takes my eyes about a minute to adjust to the dingy area, but soon I see Tim and the young man waving at me as if they've found the walls bleeding. I approach them and notice old man Robert Salter laying on his back on a bed of cardboard boxes that have been flattened to make a mattress.

The wind gusts past us and I get a cold shiver. There's an eerie whistle as bits of paper and trash blow back and forth. This would be a horrible place to call home, even without the paramedics across the street bombing you.

Tim kneels down to take a pulse and he asks me for the Airway bag. Clearly, Tim wants to work this code. The young man is beside us, all worried and nervous, hoping we can revive Robert.

I raise my hands up, "Stop, Tim! Just stop and look at what you're doing."

They both look at me like I'm some kind of horrible monster. Like I kicked Jesus in the nuts or something. Tim starts to grind his teeth, as if valuable seconds are ticking away while we deliberate.

What they don't know, that I could tell from the second we arrived down here, was that old Robert had been dead for some time. Hours, not minutes. His eyes were slightly open, looking off into the distance at some place beyond this world. His mouth is half open as if his last word was '*oooooh*.'

And I know, beyond any fraction of an inkling of a doubt, that Robert is *dead* dead. Gone, not to return.

Tim still doesn't get it. He says, "What?"

"*Mouth*, Tim," I say. "Look at his mouth."

Tim, still kneeling over the body, he gives Robert's mouth a glance and the shock of seeing a cockroach climb out the side and crawl across his face sends him reeling backwards. He crashes clumsily into all sorts of bum trash—boxes, a shopping cart, tin cans, plastic crates.

He's going nuts, now!

His hair piece is flopping around like a loose shingle during a tornado. His pants have slid down to his thighs so that we can see that he doesn't wear underwear. Nobody should ever have to see that.

And while this numbnuts is rolling around like he's being attacked by a swarm of African killer bees, I try to explain to this young man that Mr. Salter has been *deceased* for quite some time. Not dead. You don't say dead with a concerned family member. No, the word is deceased. And you have to shake your head when you say it or it won't have the right impact. You have to give it that *how could this happen* tone.

I figure that this man and the rest of the people outside with Don, are the people that make up Robert's money-hungry family. I half expect the man to start rifling through Robert's trash, looking for something he can call a last will and testament. Probate court is going to have a fun time with this.

But if they want to talk to Robert now they're going to have to hire a good psychic, or use some kind of magic spell.

Tim seems to have regained his composure and his pants, still looking a bit shaky. I tell him to hook up the monitor and get the readings for our records. As I lead the young man out of the parking structure, Tim manages to get back on his feet and hook up the monitor.

I give Don the *no-chance* nod when we get outside and he immediately grabs for his radio. He's going to call dispatch and inform them that we'll be needing a coroner. And . . . maybe an exterminator.

The family, as they learn the news about Robert, seems to display all the characteristic emotions associated with being cheated. I know these looks because I got them from my ex-girlfriend when I got caught "cheating" on her.

As they shrug their shoulders, hiss, and stomp around, I'm picturing old man Salter laughing his ass off. The wise old smoke-eater that decided he'd had enough of his greedy, money-grubbing family had gotten the final word. The reason there were bugs crawling out of him was because he had a big openmouthed smile on his face when he died.

I didn't even know the guy, other than that one time where he talked to me for a few sober minutes on his way to the hospital. I couldn't tell you anything other than what the cops told us about him. But I know this . . . I already kind of miss him.

31
Heart of Gold

October 16th
Monday, 11:22 am...

Let me try and explain to you how much Ernie really loves us here at Metro-EMS. Despite his constant dedication to every aspect of the job of being a paramedic, despite his complete and unwavering desire to take every possible call and help as many patients as he can . . . there is more to him.

According to his wife, Penny, they were having lunch at a Cracker Barrel, when he started to feel some pressure in his chest. And being a seasoned medic, he knew exactly what that meant.

Heart attack.

He starts clutching at his chest, breathing shallowly.

"Honey," Penny said, "what's going on, are you alright?"

Between small, forced breaths he glanced around, *"Get . . . me over . . . to . . . Thirty-second . . . Street!"*

The reason for this was that they were in the west side of town. That, not coincidentally, is under the watchful eyes of Willard County Ambulance Service.

Ernie knew that if his wife called 911 from there, that the service that would answer it would be the Willard County boys. And he figured that if they did come they would handle him incompetently. But that wasn't all. He also didn't want them to get to treat him. If he was to go down, it should be a Metro-EMS unit that makes the save.

The son of a bitch was risking his life on a principle. That is how bad the Turf War had gotten. We were willing to die not to ride in a Willard County ambulance. Ernie is a soldier. A team player from start to finish.

Almost a martyr.

Penny ended up just driving him to the hospital so that we wouldn't wreck an ambulance trying to get to Ernie, which we would have.

During our runs, between Ernie and me, we had hit a horse, a deer, a Firebird, numerous light poles, three stop signs, and a dog. At one point our co-workers were stenciling black figures in the shapes of the animals and other objects we were smashing into on our lockers, just like they did in World War II on the nose of the fighter planes.

Afterwards, we found out that Ernie had a pulmonary embolism—an obstruction of a pulmonary artery or one of its branches. You can't breathe and you have intense chest pain. Since your blood can't exchange oxygen, this can kill you.

What the doctors said happened is that a small fragment of clotted blood broke free from his hand injury—where he blew a hole in his palm big enough to read through, while he was cleaning one of his pistols. That bit of clotted blood worked its way through his circulatory system until it got caught in one of the pulmonary arteries.

But you know Ernie, he didn't take even a full week off. No, he was back at it within four or five days. Penny, who was the woman to deflower Ernie, couldn't believe how adamant he was about getting back to work. And so when she was telling me this story, she asked me why anyone could want to do our job so bad that they'd risk their own lives.

I didn't really have an answer that would make sense. My answers would be: driving as fast as you can, and picking up chicks who are dazzled by the fact that you save lives. Hero, manly stuff.

But Ernie's answer would be different than mine. He'd tell you it was only about one thing . . . saving lives. He didn't care about the fast driving. He was too scared to look girls in the eye, much less use his uniform and status to get laid. Ernie is the kind of pure, honest soul that really does good deeds just because they're the right thing to do.

He doesn't drink. I doubt he's ever been high. He'd *never* do a bunch of coke and bang two nurses while on duty.

He doesn't look like it, his gut and rolls hanging out from his belt, but he's a hero. Ernie is the real deal. Probably the closest thing to an angel any of us will ever know.

And if I ever go down, I hope he's the guy who answers the call.

32
THE PERFECT MOMENT

October 24th
Tuesday, 10:39 am . . .

"Springfield Dispatch to Metro-EMS . . . we have a miscarriage, eight-o-one Furnace Road. Fire department is en route."

Ernie and I are waiting for a call. We've been watching a *Married with Children* marathon and we're about to take hostages we're so bored.

Don just gives us the finger wave and we head toward the unit. We might have to control bleeding, so we'll need to bring the Trauma pack. We also might have some issues with the place in which we're going. Furnace Road might as well lead to the gates of hell. It's the kind of place where the muggers mug other muggers.

We hear our supervisor volunteering Ernie and me to the call, *"Metro-EMS to Springfield Dispatch . . . Metro-three is en route."*

As we get near the unit Ernie gives me that questioning look, as if I might want to drive. He's recently backed into a stop sign and I've been giving him relentless guff about it ever since.

"Me or you?" he asks as he opens the driver's door.

"Can you be trusted?" I say with a grin.

"Probably not."

I nod as I head to the passenger side, "You are ready, grasshopper."

We get in, light 'em up, and scream out of there like somebody might be dying. And truth is, there probably is. That's one of the things about my job. Every shift, no matter what time of day, or week, or month, or year, people are on their way out.

Every time we arrive on a scene, somebody is playing tug-of-war with the Grim Reaper and it's pretty much just us trying to thwart his efforts. The part of town we're going to, a "miscarriage" could be just about anything.

On more than one occasion we've been called to the scene of one thing, only to find out that the actual injury was completely different. All we really have is what dispatch gives us. Two or three static-laden sentences.

That's it.

Whatever the callers tell the dispatch, that's what we get. So everything is always a bit of a surprise if it turns out to be exactly what dispatch says it is. Every call is a dice roll.

It takes us seven minutes to get to Furnace Road, and we pull up to a two-story house. It's a white, wood-sided house. It's old. Older than black and white television. Older than your grandparents. And there was a musty smell.

I park behind the firetruck, and Ernie and I quickly jump out. We grab the Airway bag, the Trauma pack, and the Birthing kit. Why we brought the Birthing kit is because Ernie thought it couldn't hurt. Especially since we're supposed to be here to deal with a miscarriage.

We met two firefighters at the front door and enter the house to find hardwood floors. And that was nice. Much better than dirt floors. It was a little dark, and smells like cheap candles, but I was surprised in a good way to see that there was no chainsaw in the living room.

Upon entering, the firefighters pointed me down a long hallway to a bathroom where I could see another fireman waving at me, "She's in here!"

And by *she*, he meant a *big naked fat woman with her legs spread so wide you could see inside of her.* She had a towel over the lower half of her body, but it was still grotesque.

"Just relax," I tell her as I trade places with the fireman, entering the tiny bathroom. The floor in here is plywood. Unpainted plywood. It can't be comfortable to her portly, naked legs. The fireman booked it on out of there with a quickness that let me know he was more than grateful to see us.

"I think it's comin'," she says as she swallows.

I can tell she's in pain, and horrified. Her eyes are wide and scared; sweat soaking her hair and face. And she's fidgeting with her hands. I kneel down between her legs.

"Ma'am, can you tell me what's going on?"

"It's coming! It's coming!"

Frantically, I lift the towel to see what's going on. I don't know if she's hemorrhaging to death, or passing a watermelon, or what. Well, I squint at something that catches me by surprise. I see the top of a baby's head!

"We're delivering!" I yell to Ernie, who is right behind me, and is seeing everything that I am.

I put my cupped hands underneath the opening, hoping that the child doesn't have to land on dirty old plywood. There's so much bacteria that would find its way onto the child that it could be catastrophic. This is the absolute worst-case scenario for a delivery.

Ernie hands a sterile cloth over my shoulder. The hallway is so narrow, and the bathroom so tiny, that there is only room for one of us. And really, Ernie probably couldn't have fit into the bathroom, without covering his body in butter and using an hydraulic wedge.

I raced to get the cloth laid out on the plywood underneath my hands. Almost the second I got my hands back together, cupped to support the baby, it popped out!

Sploosh!

There was no warning. There was no noise or signal from her. One second I'm raising my hands, the next moment there is a tiny child in the palm of my left hand. This little baby is smaller than a toy doll. Smaller than a tennis ball.

"Ernie, I need the bulb-aspirator! Oxygen through a nasal cannula for blow-by. I need a blanket. Towels for the baby. I need the umbilical cord scissors and clamps," I say rapidly.

Now there's tools and equipment flying in every direction as he rifles through the Birthing kit and the Airway bag. "I'm working on it!" he barks as he gets the gear together.

In seconds, he starts handing my requests over my shoulder. The first thing he gives me is the bulb aspirator. What I did then was to suction out the baby's mouth and then nose. And this was a bit of a trick because the baby is balancing in my left hand.

Handling this newborn is like holding a dandelion. Everything you do has to be supremely delicate and deliberate. I have to get this kid breathing, but I can't rush it. It's important the order in which you perform the suction.

Mouth first, nose second.

And the reason for this is that babies have a sniffing reflex which causes them to take a deep sniff whenever their nose is touched. So if you don't clear all the gunk out of their mouth first, they might aspirate all that crud.

Right away the baby took its first breath. That old wives tale about giving a newborn a slap on the back is bunk. And dangerous. You *never* slap a newborn child. If the child needs some stimulation to breathe you can tap your fingers lightly on its feet.

Anyway, when I lifted the child and it took that magical first breath, it turned from a purplish-red to a soft pink color. It was like humanity and life were breathed into him with that first gasp. A million words could be jammed into that one second. All the emotions possible, I felt them in the space of a breath.

And as incredible as this moment was for me, this child looked to be experiencing it differently. He seemed perturbed. Angry, even.

His eyes were narrow as I dried his body off with a blue sterile surgical towel. He didn't so much cry as complain. I almost expected him to glance back at his sweating mountain of a mother and say, "I waited all this time, and this is what I get? Are you kidding me?"

The entire time I am cleaning and delicately blotting the tiny child, Ernie is screaming behind me all of the neo-natal protocols, algorithms, and modalities that we need to be following. Delivering a baby is the easy part. You just need a catcher's mit. But caring for if afterward, especially a baby born premature like this one, is a formidable task.

Premature babies have under-developed lungs and they need oxygen and warmth as quickly as possible.

Slithering down my shoulder like a snake is the oxygen tube that Ernie is carefully feeding me. I administer the oxygen by utilizing the *Blow-by* method —holding the oxygen tube away from, and perpendicular to, the newborn's mouth. This allows him to take the clean air without the pressure exerted by the tube going directly into his mouth.

The entire time we're doing this the mother is freaking completely out. She's pulling a Tim! She claims that she thought she was having a miscarriage, not a baby. She says she didn't even know she was pregnant. And I was too busy to ponder that part of her rambling. Though I can't imagine how you'd not remember the conception.

"Well," I tell her, "you have a little boy. But as soon as we're ready we're going to have to take your baby to the hospital. He's very small and needs attention immediately."

Ernie slides two plastic clamps over my shoulder. And with my free hand I attach the two clamps on the umbilical cord, about a foot away from the baby, an inch apart. Then I gnaw it off with my teeth and spit the leftover chunks of flesh over my shoulder at Ernie.

Just kidding.

Anyway, I used the surgical scissors from the Birthing kit to cut between the two clamps. The mother's end of the cord I wrapped in surgical towels and set higher than her heart to prevent bleeding. I then have her close her legs—to prevent bleeding, to delay the delivery of the placenta, and to keep us from gagging.

There is another ambulance on the way, and they'll have to deliver the placenta. They'll use the placenta for blood tests and various gourmet soups. Anyway, they have to have the placenta.

For us, it's urgent to take the child to the hospital as soon as we possibly can.

I keep the child's end of the umbilical cord sticking up above his little body, surrounded by surgical towels. Ernie hands me an emergency heat blanket—those foil-looking blankets—to wrap around the child. We have to retain as much heat as possible.

As I stand up, I yell, "Ernie!"

He grabs the oxygen bottle, and whatever he can in the other arm, and we make a beeline to the unit, leaving the mother in the capable hands of the firefighter who had been with her when we arrived. He's also a trained paramedic so she should be fine.

I've got the towel-wrapped child cradled between my arms as we head down the long dark hallway, out the door, and to the ambulance.

While we're loading up into the back of the unit, one of the firefighters is sliding in behind the wheel. Ernie cranks up the heater and I sit in the stretcher, the baby still in my arms. And the kid is just too small for anything else. There's no equipment we carry appropriate to handle a baseball-sized baby.

Once we're on our way to the hospital I hook the baby up to the Pulsoximetry unit—measures oxygen saturation and pulse rate—by attaching a small band-aid looking lead to the child's toe. As we do this I glance to the monitor and see that we're getting a good reading.

"He's pinking up!" I say enthusiastically.

The baby is small, but he is doing good considering the circumstances. He's got an APGAR score of 10. APGAR is Appearance, Pulse, Grimace, Activity, and Respiration. All of these traits are measured by a series of tests that we perform on the child. A 10 means he is doing well, and has the greatest likelihood of success in the environment outside the uterus.

Time floats by at a surreal pace as I study this tiny human. Before I know it we're arriving at the hospital. As we get out there is a neo-natal team waiting with an

isolette—clear plexi-glass chamber for carrying a baby
—just inside the emergency room entrance. They take
our little patient from us and begin doing all of the
wonderful and incredible things that doctors do in the
NICU (Neo-natal Intensive Care Unit).

I walk slowly out of the hospital and I see Ernie
sweating up a storm. I think it's probably Marlboro
time. I join him on the back of the unit and he's
halfway through his first cigarette.

He leans his head slowly back, then turns to me,
"You know, Danny . . . you get your stork pin, now."

The stork pin is awarded to a paramedic the first
time he delivers a baby in the field. We wear them on
our name tags like boy scout merit badges.

I just nod, getting a cigarette lit, as I lean my head
back. It's that first pull, and the instant rush of nicotine that calms me. I slowly exhale the bluish-gray
smoke through my nose as it drifts upward.

Moments later, our second ambulance skids to a
stop. The doors pop open and we watch as Don and
Brian hop out to unload the mother. They deliver her
to the emergency room and then Brian returns with the
gurney, pushing it to their ambulance. He then joins
Ernie and I, pulling off his bloody gloves and reaching
past us to a red bio-hazard trash bag.

I hand him a cigarette, Ernie reaches over to light
it, and the three of us lean back as our legs dangle
beneath us. Our thoughts are swimming in the cigarettes' smoky swirls.

I turn to Brian, "You know, Brian . . . you get your placenta pin, now." Of course, there is no placenta pin.

"Jesus Christ, that was disgusting! Did you see that lady?" Brian says, his face all bent and disgusted. "I'll never look at another vagina the same way. It was . . . it was some kind of . . . "

"I know," Ernie says, patting him on the shoulder. "I know."

Later we checked with the hospital staff. They informed us that the baby was *extremely* premature—3 months early—and weighed just under 2 kilograms. It had underdeveloped lungs and was slightly hypothermic—cold.

Four months and five pounds later the child went home with its mother. That kid is alive because of the combination of Ernie and me and the firefighters. But I was the one who first touched the new life.

I still think about that child every now and again. He's probably just getting old enough to steal cars and throw rocks at old ladies, but to me he's that delicate pink little fella taking his first beautiful breath.

Few things in my life have had a greater impact on me than that one moment.

EPILOGUE

March 11th
Monday, 1:52 am . . .

"***Springfield Dispatch to Metro-EMS . . .*** " came across the city-wide radio frequency.

Imagine falling off of a building and landing on a sharp piece of rusted iron, right through your stomach. Picture sliding your left hand across a piece of broken glass, leaving your fingers on the shiny surface as your brain tries to comprehend what happened. Ponder tripping backwards and cracking your head on the corner of the swimming pool while you're cleaning it in the dead of winter.

Try to imagine that feeling when your windshield is exploding in slow-motion, shards of jagged glass racing toward your face as your body is thrown around like a rag doll, pieces of hot metal and broken plastic twisting around you. This is my life.

" ***. . . motor vehicle accident at Twenty-Forth and Wall Street. Fire department is en route.***"

This was a particularly strange call for me because I wasn't answering it from the station, or anywhere near my ambulance. In fact, I *was* the call.

265

The motor vehicle in question is my new Ford Mustang.

The accident they're going on about is me smashing into a parked utility truck that was sitting dangerously in the middle of the road.

When I left the bar I got behind another drunk guy and we were just hauling ass through the city, making pretty good time. Down one particularly dark stretch of road he suddenly veered to the right, dodging a parked electric company truck. And I, well . . . I didn't veer so well.

And really, how could I? I was blitzed out of my mind, drunk, high on coke and *Xanax*. To be honest, I was completely out of my tits. Too many ghosts floating around in my head to do it sober. And by *it* I mean to say *living*.

Anyway, I crashed into this mysterious dark mass in the street and started seeing stars. I waited until the world stopped spinning before I regained my senses and pushed the door slowly open. Most of the work was done for me though, because the door was practically peeled off its hinges. I was greeted by a lonely, yellowish buzzing, street light.

I pulled myself out. When I got to the curb and sat down I felt the warm wetness of fresh blood on my head. I'm sure I'll find a matching pattern on the windshield or dashboard if I look.

Seconds later the driver of the car in front of me skidded to a stop and ran back to help me. As he approached he yelled, "Man . . . are you okay? That . . . I just barely missed that fucking truck myself! The son-of-a-bitch parked out in the middle of the road! How dangerous is that, huh?!"

I shrugged, *"Very?"*

He nods, looking around nervously. He glanced back and forth between me and my car. And within a minute or so we begin to hear the sirens approaching. "Hey, Man, I gotta get out of here. You *understand*, don't you!" And before I could answer he was gone.

Still numb and disoriented I see his car race off into the darkness, and I'm not sure if he was really here, or if I have a concussion and am already hallucinating. There's so much crap in my system right now, who knows.

About three minutes later an ambulance skids to a stop near me. Thank God it was one of ours. The doors pop open and wouldn't you know it . . . it's my old partner Ernie, and his new sidekick Brian. Relief spread through me in a way I can't explain.

If it was going to be anyone in the world to answer the call, the fact that it was the best paramedic that I've ever known was an extreme comfort to me.

I guess I should tell you that I was no longer working for *Metro-EMS*. I had taken a job that paid twice as much, and it had one perk that stood above all others: I didn't have to see dead bodies all the time. And really, it's hard enough to juggle an alcohol and drug addiction with life saving.

I had reached the end of my rope. Unlike Tim, I knew when to get out. They say that when you burn out, everyone around you will know it except you. And it is those closest to you who will suffer. Well, I *knew*.

I looked in the mirror one night after a long shift and I saw the guy looking back at me was pissed-off. His eyes were weary and unsafe.

That guy in the mirror was the person that everyone else sees when they talk to me. And that guy was barely holding on. I knew right then that I was finished.

Ernie and Brian followed their A-B-Cs, packaged me up—C-collar on my neck, towel rolls beside my swollen head, my body firmly strapped to the backboard—and then they got me loaded into the back of the ambulance. Brian was behind the wheel looking every bit as sinister and devious as I had remembered him.

Ernie, in the back with me, he says, "You're supposed to be on *this* side, Danny."

I smile, nod to him, and say, "Phone, Ernie. Where's my phone?"

He shuffles through my stuff and hands me the phone so that I can try and call my family. I end up calling my parents, my ex-girlfriend, my brother, my buddies, and even a neighbor, but nobody has time to meet me at the hospital . . . after a *wreck!*

Am I that big a jerk that I can total my car and the only people who care about me are the paramedics who have to do it for $8.50 an hour?

I eventually get in touch with . . . nobody. I left about 15 messages explaining my situation and how I needed a ride. But my phone wasn't *blowing-up* with people's sympathy.

Ernie put a 4-by-4 dressing on my head where I was bleeding from the windshield. He asked me about my injuries, where I was hurting, the usual questions needed to make his assessment.

I told him that my chest and stomach were in pain, probably from the seatbelt and steering wheel. And quietly we drove to the hospital. He didn't say much, all though I could tell that he wanted to. Perhaps, of all the injured people he's cared about more than he probably should have, he really felt for me. I could see it in his eyes, and the way he tried to look at anything other than me.

Ernie and I had shared a lot of time together. We had watched people die, brought them back to life, and been covered in blood. We had witnessed catastrophes together, sharing the carnage in a way that most people can't imagine. And when you do this for years and years with someone, you experience things for which there are no appropriate descriptions.

It's impossible to explain our friendship because it's measured in blood and chaos. Only occasionally, and for the briefest of moments, do we get to see anything that makes us smile.

So having me on the gurney beside him, it's hurting him much more than it's hurting me to be here.

Before I know it we're at the hospital and a cop I'm familiar with is asking me for a blood sample. I pulled a plastic bottle of Xanax out of my pocket and shook it a couple of times so that the few pills I hadn't already eaten rattled. I told him, "I don't think that will be necessary."

He understood. I didn't want him taking my blood and looking for anything else in my system. Because, believe me, there was a lot of *anything else*.

He made some scribbles on his pad and walked off. I sat there, alone, for hours. I can't tell you what I was thinking about, other than just not going to jail.

My new girlfriend arrived to my delight and horror. See, I hadn't had the nerve to call her because we had only just met and I didn't want to spook her with all this. I like her a lot, so I don't want her thinking I'm some kind of reckless junkie . . . even if *factually* I might be.

Somehow she had found out that I was here and came as quickly as the laws of physics would allow. She's saving me. In more ways than one. With all of my family and friends ignoring me, she was the only one that came to my aid. No flesh or blood or long-time friends . . . just her.

I told myself right then and there that I was going to marry her.

And I did.

My old supervisor Don, he came by to see me with the other guys. Don still works for Metro-EMS. I saw him on the news a few years back helping out after Hurricane Katrina. He's still a supervisor, and there still hasn't been a big enough shock to get anything more out of him then a *shooooo*.

Tim eventually capitulated to all of our pressure and quit working as a paramedic. He actually gave *me* as his reason for resigning. He took his military retirement and went back to driving dump trucks full time. As far as we know, he's still a numbnuts, puke-faced dildo who has a hairpiece older than Fidel Castro.

Patients are alive today, that might not have been if Tim had answered their calls.

Brian went on to become a full-time paramedic with Metro-EMS. He was also part of the help effort during Hurricane Katrina. I hear that he's become an exceptional paramedic, but that he has been reprimanded on at least four different occasions for dry-ice bombing incidents. Nothing formal, though, because they could never directly link him to the attacks.

Ernie still works for Metro-EMS, carrying on the legacy. He's got a strong heart, several children, a wife who could stop traffic with her face, a glove-box full of Metro-EMS stickers that he's still rumored to be placing on Willard County Ambulance vehicles, and a fat little dog that looks just like him.

If you ever get messed-up in Springfield, hope to God that these guys answer the call. You'll be in good hands.

Oh, I should tell you about Megan and Heather. You know, the little nurse vixens that represent everything wonderful about the craft. Well, Heather moved north to take care of her father. He was diagnosed with cancer and needed special attention.

In a tragic note, Megan died suddenly under rather curious circumstances. Her death is still being investigated at this time. She was so polite and caring to everyone, and such a good nurse, that I can't imagine her being involved in anything untoward. She was one of the nicest, and most charismatic women I ever met, and we all miss her.

And lest we not forget Mr. Billy Angel. The once proud DEA agent who fell from grace and became the biggest system abuser the state has ever known. Remarkably, he got himself clean. For a while, anyway. He managed to move into the Soul's Harbor shelter for a couple of months. All of the workers there said that he was doing really well, and then . . . then he suddenly disappeared.

There were rumors that he was dead, frozen in the winter cold. But just when we all thought he was gone, there was a Billy sighting in Branson. Then another one in Lebanon. Then twice in Joplin around Christmas time.

A cop here or a paramedic there would claim to have given him a ride to the hospital, or to the bus station. Then he's a ghost again, until the next arrest or ambulance call. There were even rumors of another homeless riot that Billy had masterminded.

Billy Angel is more of a legend, now. A tale passed down from paramedic to EMT; from police Lieutenant to young patrolman. He's become something of bum hero, standing bigger and taller than in real life. He's our version of Elvis. Our Jimmy Hoffa.

To this day there are still Billy Angel sightings. And I kind of like the idea that he's still out there, handling dynamite, leading insurgencies, screaming out injustice for those around him who don't have the courage to raise their voices. The world needs Billy Angels. He lets us remember our own humanity.

As I look back on everything I did during my career, from my early training to my both incredible and awful experiences, my haunted nights, my drug and alcohol addiction . . . I've put it all in context. All of it, the good and the bad and the laughter and the violence and the pain, it was worth it for that one moment I had watching that impossibly small child spark to life in my left palm.

Because in that one brief, fleeting moment, on my knees in that small plywood-floored bathroom, it was perfect. And I get it. I understand why we do the things we do. I figured out why we rush through traffic to get to a scene full of pain and chaos and images that will continue to plague our nightmares for the rest of our lives.

Every one of us—the paramedics, the EMTs, the firefighters, the first responders, and even the police officers that occasionally piss us off—do the jobs we do searching for that one perfect, golden moment.

That's the frame in time that we will replay over and over whenever we need some kind of validation. An explanation. Some *reason* for doing what we did.

In those hours between dusk and dawn when I'm alone and the thought of a drink or a line starts to creep into the back of my mind, I fight it back with that little baby, and that first breath it took.

That one perfect moment in time, *that* is my shelter.

My Soul's Harbor.

Nicholas Black & Ian Federov

SOUL'S HARBOR PROJECT

We know there are thousands of you out there who have interesting stories and experiences to share. Please join us on-line, post your stories, and tell us what you think.

We all learn from each other. Especially in the emergency medical field, where experience is our teacher.

Please visit us at:

www.SoulsHarborProject.com

Rights Available:

This is a self published work. At this time all rights are available. If you know of a charitable organization that might benefit from this book, or have any rights queries, please contact Jill Falter or Leslie at:
info@SoulsHarborProject.com

Information pertaining to this or any other issue can be sent to:
support@SoulsHarborProject.com

Acknowledgments:

This book—from the first letter to the last period—was a massive group effort by a bunch of people who know nothing about the publishing industry. But we read a lot of books and figures, hey, how hard could it be to write a book? Well, pretty hard, actually.

There are certain people in my group of friends, who showed a nearly tireless resolve in helping me edit and re-edit . . . and *re*-edit. Among them are Hank *"The Saint"* Day, Mark R. Vandeveegaete, Robert Salter, John Farlow, Rodney Starling, and Eddie Spykes, and Johnny "Shane" Wright, and Onofre "The Man" Guerra.

To Jordan Abernathy, who edited our sludge and turned it into something intelligible

Jill and Hal Falter have also been instrumental in this project getting produced. They read all my stuff when it was ugly, and told me so. They were, in fact, the only support I had from the outside, who urged that this book get published.

And finally, for Leslie, who brought this whole thing together.

Glossary of Medical Terms

Adrenaline—also called *Epinephrine.* May be injected into the hearts of victims of cardiac arrest to stimulate heart activity. It also dilates the bronchioles and in this way is an aid to respiration for asthma sufferers. Epinephrine is also useful in acute allergic disorders, such as drug reactions, hives, and hay fever.

Ambulance—a vehicle equipped for transporting the injured or sick.

APGAR—Appearance, Pulse, Grimace, Activity, Respiration. A qualitative measurement of a newborn's success in adapting to the environment outside the uterus.

A newborn infant is evaluated one minute and five minutes after birth. Five signs are assessed: heart rate, respiratory effort, muscle tone, reflex irritability, and skin color. Medical students memorize these signs by using the mnemonic of Virginia Apgar's name: *a*ppearance, *p*ulse, *g*rimace, *a*ctivity, and *r*espiration. A score of 0, 1, or 2 is assigned to each component. Usually, the higher the total score, with 10 being the maximum, the better the infant's condition. If the infant's total score is less than 7, it is reevaluated ever 5 minutes until 20 minutes have passed or until two successive scores of 7 or greater are obtained.

Albuterol Sulfate—a bronchodilator that relaxes smooth muscle surrounding the bronchi constriction and opens the airways.

Alveoli—any of the small air spaces in the lungs where carbon dioxide leaves the blood and oxygen enters it.

Atropine—poisonous, crystalline substance belonging to a class of compounds known as alkaloids and used in medicine. It is used to jumpstart the heart in emergency medicine.

BVM (*Bag Valve Mask*)—hand squeezable device used to fill the lungs with oxygen. Takes the place of mouth-to-mouth resuscitation.

Cardiac Monitor—electronic device to measure and assess cardiac rhythm. See *Lifepack-10*.

Carpuject—pre-filled medication syringe; for one-time use.

Cocaine—recreational vehicle for *Medic-13*. Cocaine acts as an anesthetic because it interrupts the conduction of impulses in nerves, especially those in the mucous membranes of the eye, nose, and throat. More importantly, cocaine when ingested in small amounts produces feelings of wellbeing and euphoria, along with a decreased appetite, relief from fatigue, and increased mental alertness.

    When taken in larger amounts and upon prolonged and repeated use, cocaine can produce depression, anxiety, irritability, sleep problems, chronic fatigue, mental confusion, paranoia, and convulsions that can cause death.

Code—any of a number of cardiac arrests. Cessation of heart function such as Myocardial Infarction, congested heart failure, etc.

Code Blue—medical code used to signify a cardiac emergency. Often, in a hospital or emergency medical environment, a call such as, "*Dr. Blue, Dr. Blue!*" will signify that there is a Code, or a cardiac emergency, followed by instructions on where the *Code team* should converge.

Demerol—also called **Meperidine**. A synthetic drug used in the treatment of moderate to severe pain. It is an opioid analgesic, and thus its effects on the body resemble those of opium or morphine, one of opium's purified constituents.

    It can be administered orally, in a tablet or liquid form, or by way of intramuscular or subcutaneous injection. Its effects are felt within 15 minutes, and may last from 3 to 5 hours. **Demerol** is highly addictive; however, its side effects tend to be less severe than those of morphine, making it a preferable choice in many situations.

Dopamine—also called *Hydroxytyramine,* a nitrogen-containing organic compound formed as an intermediate compound from dihydroxyphenylalanine (dopa) during the metabolism of the amino acid tyrosine. It is the precursor of the hormones epinephrine and norepinephrine. **Dopamine** also functions as a neurotransmitter—primarily by inhibiting the transmission of nerve impulses—in the *substantia nigra, basal ganglia,* and *corpus striatum* of the brain.

EKG—The electrocardiogram (ECG) is a graphic recording of the electrical activity of the heart detected at the body surface and amplified. For many years it was called an **EKG** after the German *Elektrokardiogramm.* Electrodes to record the electrical activity of the heart are placed at 10 different locations, one on each of the four limbs and six at different locations on the anterior chest wall. 12 different leads, or electrical pictures, are generated, each having its own normal configuration.

EMT (Emergency Medical Technician)—performs basic life-support skills both in the field and in the hospital environment. Entry level for emergency medical practitioners.

Endotracheal Tube—the rigid tube inserted into the trachea to insure a clear pathway for oxygen. Used for unconscious patients.

Epinephrine—also called *adrenaline* and *noradrenaline.* **Epinephrine** may be injected into the hearts of victims of cardiac arrest to stimulate heart activity. It also dilates the bronchioles and in this way is an aid to respiration for asthma sufferers. **Epinephrine** can be useful in acute allergic disorders, such as drug reactions, hives, and hay fever.

Fast-patch—highly adhesive pads used to deliver shock from defibrillator devices such as the *Lifepack-10* and subsequent models. They are placed on the lower left and upper right portions of the chest, to create an arc of electricity across the heart.

Gurney—a wheeled cot or stretcher used for transporting patients from the field to the hospital.

Intubation—the introduction of an endotracheal tube into a hollow organ, such as the trachea, to aid in breathing.

Larnygoscope—an instrument for examining the interior of the larynx.

Lidocaine—a crystalline compound $C_{14}H_{22}N_2O$ that is used in the form of its hydrochloride as a local anesthetic and as an antiarrhythmic agent. **Lidocaine** produces prompter, more intense, and longer lasting anesthesia than does procaine (*Novocaine*).

Lifepack-10—a type of cardiac monitor developed by the company *Physio Control*. It can assess cardiac rhythm, act as defibrillator, as well as a pacer.

Monitor—electronic device to measure and assess cardiac rhythm. Also called **Cardiac Monitor.** See also *Lifepack-10.*

Morphine— a bitter crystalline addictive narcotic base $C_{17}H_{19}NO_3$ that is the principal alkaloid of opium and is used in the form of a soluble salt (as a hydrochloride or a sulfate) as an analgesic and sedative.

   It also has a calming effect that protects the system against exhaustion in traumatic shock, internal hemorrhage, congestive heart failure, and debilitated conditions (as certain forms of typhoid fever). It is most frequently administered by injection to ensure rapid action, but it is also effective when given orally.

Neo-Natal—medical term for *newborn babies.*

Oral Airway—simple airway adjunct utilized for quick airway access. Curved, hard-plastic tube used to depress the tongue and establishes an airway until the endotracheal tube is inserted. A basic life-saving tool found in the Airway bag.

Oximeter—an instrument used for measuring continuously the degree of oxygen saturation in the circulating blood.

Oximetry—a measurement of the degree of oxygen saturation of the cir culating blood found by using an **Oximeter**. See also *Pulsoximeter*.

Paramedic—health-care workers who provide clinical services to patients under the supervision of a physician. The term generally encompasses nurses, therapists, technicians, and other ancillary personnel involved in medical care but is frequently applied specifically to highly trained persons who share with physicians the direct responsibility for patient care. This category includes nurse practitioners, physician's assistants, and emergency medical technicians.

PEA (*Pulseless Electrical Activity*)—cardiac electric activity in a heart that doesn't result in a pulse. No blood flow is created from the heart.

Pulseless V-tach—the state of being in ventricular tachycardia without a pulse. May occur during cardiac arrest.

Pulse Oximeter—type of **Oximeter** that checks both pulse and oxygen saturation.

PVC (*Premature Ventricular Contractions*)—abnormal firing of the ventricles that cause decreased cardiac output.

Pumper—firetruck equipped with a giant water tank. Make up the majority of fire department fleets. An all-purpose fire vehicle.

Sinus Rhythm—the rhythm of the heart produced by impulses from the sinus node. Typically, a cardiac rhythm denoting normal cardiac function.

Sinus Tachycardia—relatively rapid heart action whether physiological (as after exercise) or pathological.

SRT—Special Response Team. A police unit similar to SWAT.

SVN Nebulizer—medical device used to deliver medication in in a fine spray. One example would be the administration of Albuterol Sulfate during an asthma attack.

Unit—used to refer to the ambulance, rig, or truck.

Valium—also known as *Diazepam*. A tranquilizing drug used in the treatment of anxiety and as an aid in preoperative and postoperative sedation. Is also used to treat skeletal muscle spasms.

V-fib *(Ventricular Fibrillation)*—very rapid irregular contractions of the muscle fibers of the heart resulting in a lack of synchronism between heartbeat and pulse.

V-tach *(Ventricular Tachycardia)*—an abnormally fast heart rate in which the atria failed to fire. Results in insufficient or cessation of blood flow throughout the body.

Xanax—also called *alprazolam*. Drug in the benzodiazepine family, effective in relieving anxiety, and superior to barbiturates because of the reduced dangers they present of tolerance and addiction, and because they are much less likely to injuriously depress the central nervous system when used at high doses. They also require a much smaller dosage than do barbiturates to achieve their effects.

*Note to reader: We used our knowledge and various medical resources as well as the *Encyclopaedia Britannica* to produce this glossary. For a more in-depth look at any or all of the above terms, please consult a current medical practitioner and or recent medical resources. Local Protocols will override all other medical directives.

www.SoulsHarborProject.com

CPSIA information can be obtained at www.ICGtesting.com
Printed in the USA
BVOW071958161111

276292BV00001B/2/P